Hypnotherapy Explained

Hypnotherapy Explained

ASSEN ALLADIN

Adjunct Assistant Professor
Foothills Medical Centre and Department of Psychiatry and
Psychology
University of Calgary Medical School, Canada

Forewords by

MICHAEL HEAP PhD

Past President, British Society of Experimental and Clinical Hypnosis
Clinical/Forensic Psychologist
Wathwood Hospital, Rotherham

and

CLAIRE FREDERICK MD

Past Editor, *American Journal of Clinical Hypnosis*
Distinguished Consulting Faculty
Saybrook Institute of Graduate Studies and Research
San Francisco, California

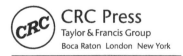

CRC Press
Taylor & Francis Group
Boca Raton London New York

CRC Press is an imprint of the
Taylor & Francis Group, an **informa** business

CRC Press
Taylor & Francis Group
6000 Broken Sound Parkway NW, Suite 300
Boca Raton, FL 33487-2742

CRC Press is an imprint of Taylor & Francis Group, an Informa business

No claim to original U.S. Government works

Visit the Taylor & Francis Web site at
http://www.taylorandfrancis.com

and the CRC Press Web site at
http://www.crcpress.com

British Library Cataloguing in Publication Data

A catalogue record for this book is available from the British Library.

ISBN-13: 978 1 84619 119 0

Typeset by Pindar New Zealand (Egan Reid), Auckland, New Zealand

Contents

Foreword by Dr. Michael Heap

It must be almost 30 years since I met Assen Alladin. We were both clinical psychologists and at that time the British Society for Experimental and Clinical Hypnosis was being established, the main impetus being that there was no existing hypnosis society for health service professionals in the UK that would admit psychologists. It was therefore very useful to have Dr. Alladin on board.

In the 1980s Dr. Alladin made two great contributions to clinical hypnosis, the first being a carefully designed project on its efficacy in the treatment of migraine. Over the years I have taught hypnosis to many clinicians and I rarely omit reference to this work, particularly the detailed protocol that Dr. Alladin found to be the most effective treatment.

Dr. Alladin's second contribution arises from his having the advantage of a very thorough grounding in cognitive therapy. He has thus been able to establish a treatment protocol for depression which he calls 'cognitive hypnotherapy' and which augments a well-planned course of cognitive behavior therapy with hypnotic procedures. I attended his first training workshop on this in Manchester, England, and still have the handouts. They have (with Dr. Alladin's kind permission) proved invaluable on the training courses with which I have been involved.

Soon after this, we in the UK suffered the loss of Dr. Alladin to our colleagues in Canada. Since then he has become a well-respected international authority on clinical hypnosis and my UK colleagues and I are regularly pleased to renew our acquaintance with him at meetings of the International and European Societies of Hypnosis.

I recall Dr. Alladin once making the very telling point that, unlike the major schools of therapy, hypnosis itself does not usually provide a theory or explanation of the conditions that it is used to treat. More problematically, often the foundations of hypnotic treatment are not informed by any well-accepted model of psychopathology, and practitioners do not always base their ideas about hypnosis on a modern, evidence-based understanding of human psychology.

The reader will find that such criticisms do not apply to the present volume.

Dr. Alladin's formula is to provide up-to-date knowledge of each condition to be treated, a model of hypnosis that is supported by modern research findings, and a sound rationale for how the latter may be applied to the former for the benefit of the patient.

This approach is illustrated by his development of cognitive hypnotherapy for depression. He makes the concept of dissociation central to his model of depression, and bases his understanding of the mechanisms of hypnosis on the neodissociation theory of Ernest Hilgard. This combination provides a rationale for the application of hypnosis to depression, but still within a cognitive behavioral framework. Moreover, certain features of depression can be construed in terms of hypnotic theory, notably the idea of depressive ruminations as a form of (negative) self-hypnosis.

Hypnotherapy Explained is not one of the many 'how to do it' guides that repeat everything that has gone before (including much of what does not bear repeating). It is a disciplined, well-researched and up-to-date account of how hypnosis can be effectively applied to ease human distress. I would not say it is only for the beginner: I am sure that experienced practitioners have much to gain from every chapter of the book.

Michael Heap PhD
Past President of British Society of Experimental
and Clinical Hypnosis
Clinical/Forensic Psychologist
Wathwood Hospital, Rotherham
September 2007

Foreword by Dr. Claire Frederick

For many years I was one of those physicians who entertained deep prejudice and disdain for the use of hypnosis in my clinical practice. As with all prejudice, my views on hypnosis were the result of sublime ignorance and the entertainment of popular, inaccurate myths and stereotypes. It would have been wonderful to have had the opportunity to access *Hypnotherapy Explained* when I was in medical school or residency training. Neither I nor most of my colleagues had been exposed to the medical uses of hypnosis in our training. Nor had we been disabused of the multitude of myths and misconceptions that surround hypnosis. My lack of accurate information held me back from bringing to my clinical work the treasure chest of hypnotic enhancement I can now provide.

The fields of clinical and experimental hypnosis not infrequently come up against barriers of closely held myth and misunderstandings among the scientific community and healthcare givers. This is true despite the American Medical Association's endorsement of clinical hypnosis in 1959 and its recommendation that hypnosis be taught in every medical school and appropriate graduate programs. Unfortunately, the professional who fails to learn the scientific facts about hypnosis may find him/herself relying on literature and movies as well as the antics of stage hypnotists as measures of the value of an important facilitator of healing. For the many patients who can benefit from hypnosis, it is indeed a tragedy that hypnosis has been so marginalized in the clinical sciences.

The history of science can be viewed through many lenses. From one perspective it appears that the applications of science can only progress when erroneous belief systems are dissolved. These belief systems usually represent the science of the earlier times in which they originated. For example, the textbook *Malleus Maleficarum (The Witches' Hammer)* was used to 'scientifically' identify the witches who needed to be burned for the safety of all. Many of these unsubstantiated – but tightly held – belief systems have been overriding sources of pain, illness and failures in growth and exploration in the history of the world. It must be emphasized that it is never only the lay person who holds such untenable beliefs. For example, Semmelweiss was thought to be insanely obsessed when he correctly insisted that puerperal fever could be avoided if hospital personnel simply washed their hands after seeing patients.

Hypnotherapy Explained brings to hypnosis the lenses of science and reason. It allows the professional to look at hypnosis from several theoretical perspectives, and it presents the research that 'good theories' generate. Dr. Assen Alladin asks the reader to take a serious look at the current, heavily researched science of hypnosis, and introduces working definitions of the hypnotic state that are essential. The professional who works through this disciplined review then moves on to a cornucopia of clinical information about hypnosis, which includes such topics as how to facilitate trance, how it can be used, and the nature of the universal effects of trance.

Hypnotherapy Explained takes its reader into the relationship of science and hypnosis. It fills a void in hypnosis education as no other book does. It is for the scientifically curious, for the clinician who wants to be able to help patients use their internal resources to a greater extent, and especially for those who wish their patients to be less dependent and more inclined and able to become involved in self-care.

This book, which is destined to be a classic in the field, is distinctive in several ways. Its approach is stringently scientific and exceedingly well referenced. There is a high degree of integration of basic science, clinical science and hypnotic technique. The reader is given bases for using hypnosis with a variety of clinical conditions. However, there is also room for explanations of empirical bases for integrating hypnosis into treatment.

Another of its unique characteristics is its unusual degree of balance. The world of scientific hypnosis is a large one, which encompasses many opinions and approaches. Dr. Alladin presents many of these in an even-handed manner. This book is also exceptional in the way it guides clinicians to do actual research as they work with their patients and to join the clinical community in its search for practice-based therapies. Finally, it is creative and warmly human. Those who know little or nothing about hypnosis could find no better introduction; those who know a great deal will find no better refresher.

Claire Frederick MD
Past Editor, *American Journal of Clinical Hypnosis*
Distinguished Consulting Faculty
Saybrook Institute of Graduate Studies and Research
San Francisco, California
September 2007

Preface

The bimonthly paper *Frontlines*, published by the Calgary Health Region, recently printed several Psychological Health Facts:* (1) a 29-year study of 7000 California adults published in 1992 found that those who were isolated and depressed had four times the risk of dying as those who were not; (2) patients with psychological disorders have on average double the number of visits to their primary care physicians as those without; (3) a 1991 study that followed mastectomy patients for 15 years found the best predictor of death from any kind of cancer recurrence was psychological response three months after surgery; (4) stress plays a role in the development and course of multiple sclerosis; (5) depressed men with HIV had a sharper decline in CD4+ cells than those who were not; (6) stress impedes the immune response to infections, increases the risk of catching a disease, prolongs the illness and worsens the risk for infection later; and (7) cognitive behavioral therapy for hostility resulted in reduced blood pressure, fewer and shorter hospital stays and significantly lower medical costs in patients with coronary heart disease.

Being a clinical psychologist I was not surprised by the report and I firmly believe in the opening sentence of the article: 'There is hardly a single ailment that can't be at least partly assuaged by paying attention to the psychological side'. This belief is based not just on my clinical training but also on my cultural heritage. During my training in clinical psychology I developed an interest in the bio-psychosocial nature of illness and became very aware of the psychological consequences of medical and psychiatric conditions. I therefore regard psychological intervention to be a very important adjunctive component in the management of both medical and psychiatric disorders.

My approach to illness and healing is also influenced by my upbringing. I was brought up on the island of Mauritius (in the Indian Ocean, about 1100 miles from the east coast of South Africa) where, on numerous occasions, I witnessed people walking on fire without fear and burning, and some people piercing their cheeks and tongues with skewers without pain or bleeding. And

---

* February 20, 2007, Issue 176; www.calgaryhealthregion.ca

the most amazing thing was that there was instant healing when the skewers were removed from the cheeks and tongue. Some of my friends who went through these religious rituals were in the taverns in the afternoon drinking rum and there was no sign of lesions in their cheeks or tongue.

I became fascinated with these religious phenomena and wanted to know more about them from a scientific perspective rather than dismissing them as unreal or fake. I reasoned that if we can understand how these people are able to control their fears, pain, bleeding and rapid healing, we will be able to apply this understanding to reducing pain and distress and promoting healing in patients suffering with various medical and psychological conditions.

In my search for an answer I stumbled on hypnosis in 1974 at the University of London, while I was a psychology undergraduate. The British Society of Experimental and Clinical Hypnosis (BSECH) was newly formed and met monthly at Birkbeck College, University of London. I became actively involved and served as Secretary for the Manchester Division of BSECH for many years. I discovered that hypnosis provided a scientific context for both studying and producing some of the phenomena I observed as a child. I was amazed that hypnosis could readily produce significant physiological, behavioral, emotional and cognitive changes, and that some people can undergo painless surgery under hypnosis without the aid of chemical anesthesia. I realized that hypnosis can serve as a powerful psychological intervention, and ever since I qualified as a clinical psychologist in 1983 I have been using hypnosis as an adjunctive procedure in my clinical practice.

Although my clinical training was significantly influenced by cognitive behavior therapy (CBT), and no doubt CBT is one of the most effective forms of psychotherapy, I found CBT to be limited in the sense that it is not experiential enough; the focus is more on thinking (cognitive restructuring). As a therapist I believe that people validate their reality by the way they feel and not by the way they think, and negative experience such as feeling anxious or depressed can be more effectively changed by producing an alternative (positive) experience. Whereas CBT lacked the experiential component, hypnosis focuses on producing experience. Hypnosis, too, has a major weakness – it does not provide a theory of psychopathology. Therefore I decided to combine CBT with hypnosis. As discussed in Chapters 1 and 3, hypnosis adds leverage to psychotherapy and the treatment effect increases if hypnosis is combined with CBT.

The aim of writing this book is to provide health professionals not familiar with hypnosis an introduction to clinical hypnosis. It is intended for beginners in general medicine and mental health, including postgraduate trainees in psychiatry, general practice, clinical psychology, counseling, psychiatric nursing, physiotherapy, speech therapy, and social work, and for undergraduate medical, nursing, psychology and social work students. I tried to write a book which I would have found useful when I started to learn clinical hypnosis. The book is not intended to act as a guide to the practice of clinical hypnosis, nor has it been written as a comprehensive review of the literature on clinical hypnosis. The aim is to provide readers with a rich source of ideas about how to start hypnotherapy and start thinking seriously about hypnosis as a powerful adjunct to psychotherapy and medical interventions. With this in mind, I have provided a selective summary (since the field is so wide) of the clinical application of hypnosis to general medicine and psychiatry. I have devoted two chapters (4 and 5) to describe in detail how hypnosis can be applied with two specific disorders: migraine and depression.

Although I have tried to give a clear and simple outline of the theory and practice of hypnotherapy, the book takes a scientific approach to hypnosis and hypnotherapy. It briefly reviews the scientific theories of hypnosis and provides a scientific and theoretical rationale for utilizing hypnotherapy with a specific disorder. The reader will have a clear definition of what hypnosis is, and they will have a clear understanding of the rationale for utilizing hypnotherapy with a particular disorder. The reader will also be able to grasp the empirical and theoretical rationale for integrating hypnotherapy with other forms of psychotherapy. Although the hypnotherapeutic strategies described in the book are brief, they are fairly detailed, so the reader can easily understand the components of the treatment.

The book consists of six chapters. Chapter 1 critically discusses the neodissociation theory of hypnosis and provides a working definition of hypnosis. The focus is on the neodissociation theory rather than other theories because it is the most widely accepted theory of hypnosis in the clinical domain. However, this focus does not undermine the role of psychosocial factors emphasized by the sociocognitive theories of hypnosis. In fact the book stresses the importance of the role of such psychosocial factors as compliance, positive expectancy and therapeutic alliance in the clinical setting. The chapter also reviews the strengths and limitations of hypnotherapy to provide the reader with a realistic view of the clinical potential of hypnotherapy.

Chapter 2 describes the eight stages of hypnotherapy, including preparing the patient for hypnosis, hypnotic induction, deepening of hypnosis, therapeutic utilization of hypnosis, ego-strengthening, post-hypnotic suggestions, self-hypnosis, and termination of hypnosis. This format provides a structure that can be easily followed and expanded on. The chapter also provides a contemporary framework for conducting clinical assessment within the context of case formulation. Such an approach to treatment is principle-driven, rather than delivering treatment in a hit-and-miss fashion. The chapter presents a full script for hypnotic induction, deepening and ego-strengthening, which can be easily adapted to the needs of a variety of patients.

Chapter 3 briefly reviews the application of hypnosis with five medical conditions and five psychiatric disorders. The review clearly demonstrates the effectiveness of hypnosis as an adjunct treatment with a variety of conditions.

Chapter 4 briefly reviews the theories and psychological treatment of migraine headache. The main focus is on the description of the hypnotherapy prototype for migraine. Eleven hypnotherapy components are described and illustrated by hypnotic suggestions scripts. Clinicians are encouraged to standardize these procedures and to validate the relative effectiveness of these procedures in the management of migraine.

Chapter 5 describes the circular feedback model of depression, which provides the rationale for combining hypnotherapy with CBT in the management of clinical depression. Cognitive hypnotherapy, based on the model, provides a variety of treatment interventions for depression, from which a therapist can choose the best-fit strategies for a particular depressed client. Cognitive hypnotherapy also offers an innovative technique for developing antidepressive pathways.

Finally, Chapter 6 provides information about training in clinical hypnosis and gives the addresses and web pages of various professional hypnosis organizations.

I hope this book will enable readers to feel excited about exploring the clinical effectiveness of hypnosis. Practitioners and students whose interest and training are in alleviating distress will find within the field of hypnotherapy a variety of mind–body techniques for unravelling and modifying the bio-psychosocial factors that may be causing and maintaining the symptoms.

Assen Alladin
September 2007

About the Author

Dr. Assen Alladin is a clinical psychologist and Adjunct Assistant Professor at Foothills Medical Centre and Department of Psychiatry and Psychology at the University of Calgary Medical School. He has been practicing hypnosis for over 20 years. He has been the Secretary of the British Society of Experimental and Clinical Hypnosis for many years and is currently the President of the Canadian Society of Clinical Hypnosis, Alberta Division.

Dr. Alladin has presented addresses and workshops on clinical hypnosis at national and international conferences. He is the author of the *Handbook of Cognitive Hypnotherapy for Depression: an evidence-based approach* (Lippincott Williams and Wilkins, 2007), and he has published several chapters and papers on clinical hypnosis. He is interested in the empirical validation of clinical hypnosis and the integration of hypnosis with cognitive behavior therapy. He was the 2005 recipient of the Best Research Paper from Division 30 of the American Psychological Association. He was a Fellow of the Royal Society of Medicine and Associate Fellow of the British Psychological Society.

Dr. Alladin has served as Guest Editor for Special Issues in Hypnotherapy for the *Journal of Preventive Neurology and Psychiatry* (1992) and for the *Journal of Cognitive Psychotherapy: An International Quarterly* (1994). He also served as Guest Editor for the *International Journal of Clinical and Experimental Hypnosis* for the Special Issues on Evidence-Based Hypnotherapy Practice (April and July 2007).

Dr. Alladin comes from the island of Mauritius and completed all his studies in England, initially training as a psychiatric nurse and social worker before qualifying in psychology and clinical psychology. Dr. Alladin now lives in Calgary, Alberta, Canada, and loves traveling.

Acknowledgements

I am grateful to a number of people who provided their continuing support and assistance during this project.

My wife, Naseem, kept nagging me to finish the project by the deadline. My son, Adam, constantly inspired me by inquiring about the scientific validity of hypnosis. Farrah, my daughter, expressed her pride in me writing this book.

Jim Arthurs, Unit Manager, and Dr. Michael King, Psychology Manager, from Foothills Medical Centre provided encouragement and allowed me time off to work on this project.

I would also like to thank Maggie Pettifer, Commissioning Editor, Radcliffe Publishing, for providing support and guidance. Thanks are also due to Stan Wakefield from Electronic and Database Publishing Inc. who got me involved with this project three years ago.

CHAPTER 1

Current Theories of Hypnosis

SUMMARY

This chapter reviews the neodissociation theory of hypnosis because it is the most widely accepted theory of hypnosis in the clinical domain. However, this focus on the neodissociation theory does not undermine the role of psychosocial factors emphasized by the sociocognitive theorists. Psychosocial factors can be judiciously utilized in the clinical setting to enhance compliance, positive expectancy and therapeutic alliance.

From the review of the brain-mapping studies of hypnosis and consciousness, it is apparent that it is unrealistic to expect a single physiological signature of hypnosis. The brain correlates of the hypnotic phenomena are determined by the quality (associated with imagery, relaxation or alertness) of the hypnotic induction, the trance level (hypnotic ability, degree of absorption and dissociation), and the nature (specificity and intensity of suggestions) of the hypnotic suggestions.

Just as we do not have a complete theory of hypnosis, we do not have a perfect definition of hypnosis. Several definitions are discussed, and finally a working definition of clinical hypnosis is presented. The chapter also highlights the strengths and limitations of hypnotherapy to provide the reader with a realistic view of the clinical potential of hypnotherapy.

INTRODUCTION

The aim of this chapter is to describe the neodissociation theory of hypnosis, which is one of the most dominant contemporary theories of hypnosis. Apart from having inspired – and still inspiring – extensive research, the theory provides a rationale for clinical work. Rather than reviewing the literature on the applications of hypnosis, the strengths and limitations of clinical hypnosis are reviewed to provide the reader with a critical perspective on the clinical applications of hypnosis to medicine and psychiatry. Finally, a contemporary working definition of hypnosis is provided.

Although hypnosis has existed as a treatment for medical and psychological disorders since time immemorial, as yet we do not have a clear definition or theory of hypnosis. Most of the theories advanced to explain hypnosis can be loosely classified under state and non-state, intrapersonal and interpersonal, or single and multifactor theories (Yapko, 2003).

State, *intrapersonal* and *single* theorists conceptualize hypnosis as a trance state or an altered state of consciousness (Barber 1969). The *non-state*, *interpersonal* and *multifactor* theorists, also known as *sociocognitive theorists*, suggest a social–psychological explanation of hypnosis. These theorists maintain that there is nothing unique about hypnosis and argue that most of the hypnotic phenomena can occur without a hypnotic induction or trance (Barber, 1979). The *intrapersonal* theories of hypnosis emphasize the subjective and inner states of the hypnotized person, whereas the *interpersonal* models attach more importance to the social context or relational aspects of the hypnotic interaction (Yapko, 2003). The *single* model of hypnosis stresses the importance of a single variable such as relaxation or dissociation that influences the hypnotic experience. The *multifactorial* approaches attach importance to the role of a variety of interactional forces, such as patient expectation and clinician demands, which combine to produce the hypnotic phenomena (Kirsch, 2000).

Although none of these theories have satisfactorily explained all the phenomena associated with hypnosis, the different formulations have certainly broadened our understanding of the subject. It is beyond the scope of this book to discuss the merits and controversies surrounding each theory (*see* Kallio and Revonsuo, 2003, for a review, and rejoinders in the whole issue of *Contemporary Hypnosis*, 2005; 22(1): 1–55). For the present purpose it is sufficient to restate the conclusions drawn by Rowley (1986, p. 23) from his review of the well-known theories of hypnosis 20 years ago:

None of them seem to be able to deal adequately with all the phenomena which come under the general heading of hypnosis. This is perhaps not surprising given the tremendous variety of phenomena. Accordingly the theories have different ways of dealing with this variety. Some redefine hypnosis, e.g. Edmonston (1981). Others reinterpret subjective experience, e.g. Spanos (1982) . . . Despite these inadequacies, each of the theories has something to offer, a new conceptualization of the issues, a methodological approach, a new synthesis of the evidence. Of course, in one sense it is impossible to produce a theory which is satisfactory to all researchers, for they are likely to have different criteria for evaluating theories.

A decade later, Yapko (2003, p. 61), from his review of the contemporary theories of hypnosis, came up with similar conclusions, especially when addressing the complexity and multidimensional nature of hypnosis:

> With a subject as complex as hypnosis, the inadequacy of a single theory's ability to explain the broad range of responses on so many different dimensions of experience becomes glaringly apparent. The complexities of the subject of hypnosis, and even greater complexities of the human being capable of hypnosis, are so great that it seems highly improbable that a single theory can evolve to explain its origin and character.

Academics and experimentalists have generally tended to adopt non-state, interpersonal and multifactorial views of hypnosis, whereas clinicians have taken the state, intrapersonal and single views of hypnosis, particularly the neodissociation theory of hypnosis, which is described below. However, proponents of both camps agree that hypnotic suggestions can produce altered states and that some subject variables such as co-operation (Spanos and Barber, 1974), expectations (Barber 1984, 1999), motivation (Araoz, 1981, 1985) and level of involvement in suggestion-related thoughts and images (Erickson and Rossi, 1979; Spanos and Barber, 1974) can influence the hypnotic performance.

For example, Kirsch (2005), a well-known sociocognitive theorist, points out that both state and non-state theorists agree that hypnotic suggestions can produce altered states such as amnesia, analgesia and involuntariness, although there is disagreement about whether these altered experiences depend on the prior induction of a trance state. Similarly, Spiegel (2005, p. 32), a well-known state theorist, underlines that:

> Multilevel explanations are an absolute necessity in understanding human mind/brain/body phenomena because we are both neurally-based and social creatures who experience the world in mental phenomenal terms. To choose one of these domains as the complete explanatory context is to be by definition wrong.

Clinicians, who are mainly concerned with reducing patients' distress, are not overly concerned whether hypnotic trance exists or does not exist, or whether trance induction is necessary or not necessary. To the clinicians, the clinical context and the skilful negotiation of subjects and other variables to maximize therapeutic gains are of paramount importance. Heap (1988, p. 3) regards this bidirectional relationship between the patient and the hypnotist in the clinical context as:

> An interaction between two people characterized by a number of inter- and intra-personal processes of which the 'essence of hypnosis' only forms a part, if indeed it is present at all. These processes, which are not independent of one another (and which may apply to the behaviour and experience of both the subject and the hypnotist) include the following: selective attention, imagination, expectancy, social conformity, compliancy, role-playing, attribution, usually though not necessarily, relaxation, rapport, suggestion, and hypnotic or trance experience.

Moreover, clinicians emphasize the subjectivity of hypnosis and recognize that hypnotic techniques must be individualized for the patient, which can involve drawing upon techniques from more than one theoretical model. The treatment approach described in this book utilizes different therapeutic techniques derived from diverse theoretical conceptualizations. Golden *et al.*, (1987) describe this approach as *technical eclecticism*. In this approach the clinician, in order to maximize therapeutic effects, borrows techniques freely from diverse therapeutic approaches without necessarily accepting the theories from which the techniques were derived. In this context, the therapist is more concerned with reducing the patient's level of distress rather than adhering blindly to a particular theoretical orientation.

NEODISSOCIATION THEORY OF HYPNOSIS

The neodissociation theory of hypnosis is described in detail here because it (a) has inspired extensive research, (b) provides a rationale for clinical work

(Kihlstrom, 2003; Lynn and Kirsch, 2006) and (c) continues to be one of the most influential contemporary theories of hypnosis. The focus on the neodissociation theory is not meant to discredit the contributions made by other competing or complementing theories of hypnosis. The aim here is to describe a theory that has been traditionally embedded within the clinical context. Indeed, the hypnotherapeutic techniques described in this book freely draw on other theories to enhance positive expectancy and treatment gains. For example, the *cognitive hypnotherapy* for depression described in Chapter 5 actively utilizes the subject's variables and placebo effects (emphasized in the sociocognitive theories of hypnosis) to maximize treatment gains.

Hilgard (1973, 1974, 1986) describes hypnosis in terms of *dissociation* or *divided consciousness*. Dissociation is a psychological process whereby information (incoming, stored or outgoing) is actively deflected from integration with its usual or expected associations, producing alteration in thoughts, feelings or actions, so that for a period certain information is not associated or integrated with other information in the usual manner or in a logical way (West 1967). Such an experience can be regarded to be either normal or pathological.

Ever since Janet (1907), the close relationship between hypnosis and dissociation has been established. Janet (1889) held the view that systems of ideas can become split off from the main personality and exist as an unconscious subordinated personality, but capable of becoming conscious through hypnosis. The theory was applied to hypnosis and various other normal and pathological states such as automatism, amnesia, fugues and multiple personality. Hilgard, by deriving ideas and concepts from information processing, selective attention, brain functioning and the cognitive model of consciousness, reformulated the theory in contemporary terms and called it *neodissociation theory*.

In Hilgard's reformulation, dissociation is seen as an extension of normal cognitive functioning. He posited that during ordinary consciousness information is processed at a number of levels by a hierarchy of cognitive operations and controls. Ordinarily these operations are integrated, but during hypnosis or dissociation the integration decreases, and certain aspects of experiences may not be available to consciousness. Within this model, dissociation or hypnotic involvement is not seen as an either/or phenomenon, but a cognitive process ranging on a continuum from minor or limited to profound and widespread dissociation. Hilgard also considered the role of *self* and *will* when formulating his neodissociation theory of hypnosis. He maintained that hypnosis and other dissociative experiences all involve some degree of loss of voluntary control or *division of* control (e.g. a hypnotized subject experiencing eye catalepsy may not be able to open his or her eyes when challenged to do so).

The neodissociation theory proposes that an individual possesses a number of cognitive systems, hierarchically arranged, with a central control structure (*executive ego*) and multiple superordinate and subordinate structures, each with its own input and output connections with the world. Although the executive ego is normally in control, the other structures can take over as a result of hypnotic-type suggestions or other similar procedures or situations. In other words, hypnosis or other similar procedures have the effect of dissociating these systems from one another, and as a result some of these systems can be taken out of awareness or consciousness. A hypnotized individual may thus report feeling no pain, but the 'hidden observer', which is the name Hilgard gives to the cognitive system which is aware of what is going on, may report feelings of pain.

To investigate the *hidden observer* effect empirically, Hilgard (1986) utilized experiments involving hypnotic analgesia and automatic writing. This effect was demonstrated by suggesting to the hypnotic subject that when a pre-arranged signal (such as the placing of the hypnotist's hand on the subject's shoulder) is given, the hypnotist will be able to contact a 'hidden part' unknown to the subject's present conscious 'part'. Hilgard claims that when this suggestion is given to responsive subjects, one is able to contact another system of control which can then speak, unaware of the normal 'waking' part, or the 'hypnotized' part. These parts are not normally aware of each other because they are separated by 'amnesic barriers'. The amnesic barriers can sometimes break down partially or completely, causing incongruities.

The automatic or involuntary nature of hypnotic responding can be easily explained by this process. For example, in automatic writing the active part that is writing is dissociated or split from the conscious part that is unaware that such an activity is taking place. Instead, the hidden observer or a covert cognitive system is aware of the automatic writing. The hidden observer can also be accessed after the termination of hypnosis by providing post-hypnotic instructions during hypnosis. The neodissociation theory proposes that when a subject is hypnotized, only some of the cognitive systems are involved, others remaining unaffected:

> Thus a person who experiences only a vague feeling of relaxation has only a very few low level cognitive systems affected. A person who experiences arm levitation and analgesia has many more cognitive systems affected. (Rowley, 1986, p. 16).

Besides hypnosis, other factors such as fatigue, stress, relaxation and daydreaming can also produce dissociation. Moreover, hypnosis can occur spontaneously, or it can be externally induced or self-induced.

Hilgard was ahead of his time in linking hypnosis with the concept of consciousness. With the recent renewed interest in the scientific study of consciousness in the areas of affective and cognitive neuroscience (e.g. Gazzaniga, 2000; Mesulam, 2000; Zeman, 2001), we have a better understanding of the relationship between consciousness and hypnosis. For example, some striking parallels have been observed in the mental processes involved in dreaming and hypnosis. Llinas and Pare (1991) observed dissociations between specific and non-specific thalamocortical systems underpinning dreaming, implying that a state of hyperattentiveness to intrinsic activity can occur without the registration of sensory input. Similarly, Furster (1995), in dreaming observed a dissociation between context/sensory input and the cognitive features of dreaming such as altered sense of time, absence of temporality, lack of guiding reality and critical judgement, anchoring in personal experience, and affective coloring. These findings led Gruzelier (1998, p. 18) to draw parallels between hypnosis and an altered state of consciousness:

> The fragmented networks activated in the dream seem to lack the associative links to a time frame, anchored as they are in the present, without time tags and references. This could equally be a description of the hypnotic state as high susceptibles experience it.

Although Hilgard's neodissociation theory of hypnosis appears logical, intuitive and subject to empirical validation, his theory is incomplete. For instance, he proposed cognitive structures to explain dissociation, but he gave little information about what happens inside them and it is not clear how many cognitive systems a person possesses and how many of these are engaged in hypnosis. However, Woody and Sadler (1998) have argued that the neodissociation theory of hypnosis is a 'good' theory despite being 'incomplete'. They believe a good theory provides a provisional framework that casts the phenomena in question in a new or distinctive light that can be subjected to empirical verification to extend our understanding of the phenomena. They believe a good theory can serve this role even if it is incomplete or has obvious areas of inadequacy. Since the neodissociation theory has generated and provoked extensive empirical research, the theory can be seen as 'quite successful' (Woody and Sadler, 1998, p. 192). Even Hilgard (1991, p. 98) openly admitted: 'I regret to leave the theory in this incomplete form, so that it is more of a promise than a finished theory'.

The neodissociation theory has also been criticized for ignoring the role of social compliance. This limitation of the theory was again readily acknowledged by Hilgard (1986), who moved towards a moderate position by using the word 'state' metaphorically to de-emphasize hypnosis as a purely special state. Moreover, some of his followers have addressed the role of social compliance in hypnosis. For example, Nadon *et al.*, (1991) have proposed an interactionist approach in which both cognitive and social factors play a part.

Some criticisms have also been levelled at the scientific validity of the hidden observer phenomenon. Although Hilgard (1986) and Watkins and Watkins (1979) have provided experimental evidence for the presence of the hidden observer (*see* Hilgard, 1986), the studies and interpretation of the hidden observer have been questioned by sociocognitive theorists. In several studies, Spanos and his colleagues demonstrated that the reports of the hidden observer varied as a function of the explicitness of instructions the subjects received about the nature of the hidden observer. For example, Spanos and Hewitt (1980) obtained reports of 'more' or 'less' hidden pain as a function of whether the subjects were told that their hidden parts would be either 'more aware' or 'less aware' of the actual amount of pain. These findings led Spanos and Coe (1992) to conclude that the hidden observer phenomenon may not be an intrinsic characteristic of hypnosis, but a social artefact shaped by subject's expectations and situational demand characteristics.

One study (Spanos *et al.*, 1984) manipulated the instructions to produce two hidden observers: one sorting memories of abstract words and the other storing memories of concrete words. This led Lynn and Kirsch (2006) to argue that the hidden observer is implicitly or explicitly suggested by the hypnotist, and hence they dubbed the hidden observer phenomenon the 'flexible observer'. However, the fact that the hidden observer reports vary with instructions does not disprove the neodissociation theory of hypnosis. On the contrary, Kihlstrom and Barnier (2005) declare that it is in the very nature of hypnosis for the hypnotized subject's behaviors and experiences to be influenced by the wording of suggestions and the subject's interpretations of them. Therefore, studies supporting the hypothesis that covert reports are influenced by suggestions are not evidence that the hidden observer is a methodological artefact, or not a reflection of the divided consciousness.

Kihlstrom and Barnier (2005) point out that researchers:

. . . with their own areas of interest and expertise, will naturally emphasize one or the other aspect of hypnosis in their work. But . . . a proper understanding of hypnosis will only come from taking the hypnotic subject's experience seriously and seeking to understand how that experience emerges from the interaction of cognitive and social processes. (p. 149)

Naish (2005) went even further to state that the hypnotized person's experience should be the main subject of research, not the behavior of the hypnotized person. He contends that proper hypnosis research should be directed at elucidating the mechanisms that bring about the hypnotic experience and not at extrapolating from simulation (using simulators) studies. He argues that studying simulators may have little to contribute to the understanding of the hypnotic phenomenon because simulators do not share their experience with the hypnotized person. He proposes that the role of simulators should be confined to studies involving spontaneous, non-suggested hypnotic behavior.

Naish believes it is perverse for critics of the neodissociation theory to ignore genuine experiences and associated cortical changes occurring in hypnotized subjects, and to simply confine the investigation to the social context of the experiment. For example, Szechtman *et al.* (1998), in their brain-mapping studies, demonstrated that when highly hypnotizable subjects were claiming to be experiencing hallucinations, the observed brain activity was extremely like that resulting from true sensory stimulation. Similarly, Kosslyn *et al.* (2000) showed that hypnotized individuals cortically responded to suggested experiences (colors) rather than to the actual stimuli in measurable ways.

Gruzelier (2005) believes that sociocognitive theorists tend to ignore these findings because of their lack of engagement with neuroscientific evidence, resulting from their pedagogical background and their lack of appreciation of the reductionist levels of neuroscientific explanation. He believes there is, for example, abundant neurophysiological and neurocognitive evidence to support the hypothesis that the anterior cingulated cortex and the left dorsolateral prefrontal cortex are involved in hypnotic analgesia. Gruzelier (2005) laments the fact that the sociocognitive theorists continue to turn a blind eye to these findings, and he is concerned that:

. . . while it is one thing to make the admission of a lack of understanding, it is quite unscientific to opine that there is no evidence for an ASC [altered state of consciousness] perspective, and to go on to attribute hypnosis to purely psychological constructs. (p. 4)

He believes it is unproductive for scientists from different theoretical backgrounds to work in isolation from each other and continue to ignore findings from opposing theoretical orientations. He claims the field of hypnosis can be easily unified through active collaboration of scientists with neurophysiological and social orientations.

Further support for the state or neodissociation theory of hypnosis comes from the research on pain and hypnosis. From his review of the recent neuro-imaging studies of the hypnotic modulation of pain, Feldman (2004, pp. 197–8) highlights several findings that elucidate the nature of hypnosis and the clinical implications for pain management.

- ○ Although the perception of pain is an integrated process, hypnotic suggestions enable subjects to distinguish between the sensory and affective components of pain.

- ○ The degree of hypnotic modulation of sensory or affective response to pain correlates with hypnotic suggestibility.

- ○ Hypnosis enables hypnotically responsive individuals to do what they cannot do in a non-hypnotic state (e.g. control the sensory aspect of pain).

- ○ Hypnosis is a more potent clinical tool for pain management than non-hypnotic approaches such as relaxation and cognitive behavior therapy.

- ○ When utilizing hypnosis for pain management, clinicians should not make the common error that pain is a purely sensory experience.

- ○ In a non-hypnotic state (e.g. distraction, relaxation) a person cannot differentiate between the sensory and affective dimensions of pain. In contrast, a person in a hypnotic state, in response to hypnotic suggestions, can not only make a distinction, but can differentially modulate sensory and affective dimensions of pain while producing corresponding differential activation of brain structures. These findings support the state theory of hypnosis.

- ○ Further support for the state theory of hypnosis is reported by Freiderich *et al.* (2001), who found that highly suggestible individuals were able to significantly lower pain, either by distraction of attention or via hypnotic analgesia, compared to the control condition. However, amplitudes of laser-evoked brain potential demonstrated that hypnotic analgesia and non-hypnotic distraction of attention involved different brain mechanisms.

○ The original proposal of the neodissociation theory that hypnotic analgesia involves the disruption or dissociation of sensory information from conscious awareness is supported empirically.

○ The recent findings provide a new hypnotic technique for moderating or facilitating dissociation from the *affective* component of pain. If an individual is unable to dissociate from the sensation of pain, especially when in severe pain, the individual may respond to suggestions of diminishing the affective component of pain. Rainville and his associates (e.g. Rainville *et al.*, 2002) have demonstrated that hypnotic suggestions can reduce distress, although the degree of pain sensation may remain unchanged.

○ Hypnotic induction and hypnotic suggestions activate different brain areas respectively (e.g. Rainville *et al.*, 2002). These findings demonstrate that hypnotic induction alone is not as powerful as hypnosis associated with specific suggestions.

○ Therefore, crafting of suggestions relevant to the nature of pain is very important.

○ The left prefrontal cortex is activated by suggestions for pain reduction. This brain area corresponds to the elicitation of positive emotional affect.

○ The above 'findings are consistent with the notion that hypnotic states are achieved through the modulation of activity within a distributed network of cerebral structures involved in the regulation of consciousness states' (Rainville *et al.*, 2002, p. 898).

ALTERED STATE OF CONSCIOUSNESS

Because hypnosis is related to the concept of consciousness, a brief description of the different states of consciousness is in order here. Ludwig (1966) defines *altered state of consciousness* (ASC) as an altered state according to subjective experience and altered psychological functioning. According to Ludwig, alteration in sensory input, physiological changes and motor activity can produce an altered state in which 'one's perception of an interaction with the external environment is different than the internal experience' (Brown and Fromm, 1986, p. 34). Tart (1975), in order to avoid the debate about whether hypnosis is or is not a state, from a clinical perspective distinguishes (a) a baseline state of consciousness (b-SOC), (b) discrete states of consciousness (d-SOC) and (c) a discrete altered state of consciousness (d-ASC).

Baseline consciousness is akin to the concept of 'cohesive self' described by Kohut (1977). Kohut defines the cohesive self as a mental and physical unit which has cohesiveness in space and continuity in time. Baseline consciousness is stabilized by a number of processes, including dealing with the variability in the environment. A *discrete state of consciousness* (d-SOC) is described by Tart (1975) as a unique and dynamic pattern or configuration of psychological structures. Although the components or subsystems of the psychological structures with a d-SOC can show some variation – as in ordinary waking state, sleep or dreaming – the overall pattern and the overall system properties remain recognizably the same. A *discrete altered state of consciousness* (d-ASC) refers to a state that is different from some baseline consciousness and forms a new system, with unique properties that have been generated as a restructuring of consciousness or reality. The word 'altered' is purely a descriptive term, carrying no values. In this sense, the hypnotic experience is seen to be generated from the internal construction of attitudes, values, motivations and expectancies. In other words, a hypnotic experience or a d-ASC is a subjective experience resulting from re-configuration or repatterning of existing resources or cognitions.

Several reviewers, such as Brown and Fromm (1986) and Rowley (1986), believe that Hilgard's theory of hypnosis meets Ludwig's and Tart's criteria for an altered state of consciousness. Hypnosis as an altered state of consciousness has been described both theoretically and experientially along the dimension of alteration in perception, cognition, awareness of one's surroundings and absorption in an unusual experience (e.g. Fromm, 1977; Gill and Brenman, 1959; Hilgard, 1977; Orne, 1959; Shor, 1959). For instance, Orne (1959), in an experiment, demonstrated the presence of 'trance logic' and negative and positive hallucinations in highly hypnotized subjects, but not in unhypnotized subjects.

The study of consciousness, unconscious processing and ASC is generating lots of interest in the neurosciences, and Gruzelier (2005) believes this is likely to herald fresh approaches to the neuroscientific understanding of hypnosis. The Altered States of Consciousness research consortium, which was formed in Germany in 1998 to study the psychobiology of ASC utilizing the latest models and methods in cognitive neuroscience, has already made an impact on the study of hypnosis and consciousness. The findings of its first six-year funded research were reported by the consortium in the *Psychological Bulletin* (Vaitl *et al.*, 2005, pp. 98–127). This paper reviewed the psychological and neurobiological investigations of consciousness and concluded that different states of consciousness are influenced by compromised brain structure, transient changes in brain dynamics such as disconnectivity, and changes in neurochemical and metabolic processes. As regards hypnosis, the review stated that 'studies suggest that hypnosis affects integrative functions of the brain and induces an alteration or even breakdown between subunits within brain responsible for the formation of conscious experience' (p. 110). Gruzelier (2005) believes that the reawakening of ASC in cognitive neuroscience will offer new perspectives on the understanding of ASC and will facilitate revisiting old considerations in a fresh way.

From these recent developments it is becoming clear that it will be unrealistic to expect a unique physiological signature of hypnosis. Since the hypnotic induction and production of the hypnotic experience/phenomenon involve a variety of multifactorial and interactional forces, different levels of the hypnotic experience may involve different parts of the brain. In other words, there is no direct neuropsychophysiological correlate of hypnosis. The neuropsychophysiological correlates of hypnosis depend on the nature and quality of the hypnotic induction and the types of suggestions and imagery used. As noted before, for example, the left prefrontal cortex, which corresponds to the elicitation of positive emotional affect, is activated by suggestions for pain reduction.

STRENGTHS AND LIMITATIONS OF HYPNOTHERAPY

Although hypnotherapy can be used as an adjunct with a variety of medical and psychological conditions, it is not a panacea for all ailments. Just like any other approaches to treatment, hypnotherapy has its strengths and limitations. Recently, Alladin (2007) reviewed the strengths and limitations of clinical applications of hypnosis, and some of these are summarized below.

Strengths of hypnosis

Adds leverage to treatment

By producing rapid and profound behavioral, emotional, cognitive and physiological changes (De Piano and Salzberg, 1981), hypnosis facilitates treatment and shortens treatment time (Dengrove, 1973).

Strong placebo effect

Most of the patients receiving hypnotherapy are self-referred or referred by other therapists or physicians, so an element of positive expectancy already exists. As the therapist gains reputation as a hypnotherapist or an expert in clinical hypnosis, not only do the number of referrals increase but also the credibility of the therapist increases. According to Lynn and Kirsch (2006, p. 31), these 'patients almost invariably hold positive attitudes and expectations about hypnosis, which makes them good candidates for hypnotic interventions'. For these patients, hypnosis acts as a strong placebo. Lazarus (1973) and Spanos and Barber (1974) have provided evidence that hypnotic trance induction procedures are beneficial for those patients who believe in their efficacy. The creative and sensitive therapist can build the right atmosphere to capitalize on suggestibility and expectation effects to enhance therapeutic gains (Erickson and Rossi, 1979).

Breaking resistance

Hypnotherapy allows the therapist the flexibility to utilize either direct or indirect suggestions. Very often patients resist direct suggestions for change. Erickson (Erickson and Rossi, 1979) utilized various indirect hypnotic suggestions to break patients' resistance. For example, he devised paradoxical instructions to minimize patients' resistance to suggestions. In the case of an oppositional (to suggestions) patient, he would instruct (paradoxically) the patient to continue to resist, as a strategy to obtain compliance.

Erickson also used 'pacing' and 'leading' strategies for reducing resistance. *Pacing* is when the therapist's suggestions match the patient's ongoing behavior and experiences. As the patient becomes receptive to pacing, the therapist can *lead* and offer more directive suggestions. For example, the therapist may pace the patient by suggesting 'as you exhale' as the patient exhales and then lead by adding 'you will begin to relax' (Golden *et al.*, 1987, p. 3).

Therapeutic alliance

Skilful hypnotic induction and repetition of positive hypnotic experience foster a strong therapeutic alliance (Brown and Fromm, 1986). When patients perceive the positive experience to be emerging from their own inner resources, they gain greater confidence in their own abilities, and this helps to foster greater trust in the therapeutic relationship.

Rapid transference

Full-blown transference can occur very rapidly, often during the initial stage of hypnotherapy, because the hypnotic experience allows greater access to fantasies, memories and emotions (Brown and Fromm, 1986). Such transference reinforces the therapeutic alliance and positive expectancy.

Relaxation response

The majority of patients treated by hypnotherapists have some element of anxiety. Due to their anxiety, anxious and agitated patients are often unable to pinpoint their maladaptive thoughts and emotions. Deep relaxation is easily induced by hypnosis, and once relaxed the level of anxiety is diminished, making it easier for patients to think about and discuss material they were previously too anxious to confront. Relaxation induced by hypnosis also reduces distraction, which maximizes the ability to concentrate, resulting in greater awareness of thoughts and feelings, and thus facilitates the ability to learn new materials.

Divergent thinking

Patients with psychological disorders, particularly depressives, tend to be convergent (narrow) thinkers. Hypnosis facilitates divergent (broader) thinking by (a) maximizing awareness along several levels of brain functioning, (b) maximizing the focus of attention and concentration, and (c) minimizing distraction and interference from other sources of stimuli (Tosi and Baisden, 1984). Because divergent thinking involves broader thinking, it increases the potential for learning alternatives.

Attention to wider experiences

In addition to convergent thinking, patients with psychological disorders and chronic medical conditions tend to selectively ruminate on certain negative feelings. Hypnosis provides a frame of mind where attention can be directed to a wider experience, such as a feeling of warmth, or feeling happy. These experiences reinforce the belief that negative experience is not permanent; it can be changed, modified and replaced by alternative feelings.

Engagement of the non-dominant hemisphere

Hypnosis provides a vehicle for direct entry into cognitive processing, such as accessing and organizing emotional and experiential information, largely served by the right cerebral hemisphere (in right-handers). By engaging the right hemisphere, the hypnotic experience is intensified, providing strong validation of reality. As humans we do not validate reality by the way we think, but by the way we feel. When an anxious patient is feeling panicky, although this may be due to irrational beliefs (e.g. 'I'm having a heart attack' when there is no evidence of heart attack), the feeling is real to the person experiencing it and thus the anxious person's reality ('There's something seriously wrong with me' or 'I can't handle the situation') is validated. The induction of an intense positive experience via hypnosis provides the validation of an alternative or positive reality. The best way to change an experience is to produce another experience. Hypnosis provides rapid induction of an alternative reality.

Access to non-consciousness processes

Various medical and psychological conditions can be caused and/or maintained by unconscious factors. Hypnosis allows access to psychological processes below the threshold of awareness, thus providing a way to explore and restructure non-conscious cognitions and experience related to the symptoms.

Integration of cortical functioning

Hypnosis provides a vehicle whereby cortical and subcortical functioning can be accessed and integrated. Since the subcortex is the seat of emotions, access to it provides an entry into the organization, processing and modification of primitive emotions.

Imagery conditioning

Because hypnosis, imagery and affect are all predominantly mediated by the same right cerebral hemisphere (Ley and Freeman, 1984), imagination is easily intensified by hypnosis (Boutin, 1978). Hypnosis thus provides a powerful modality for imagery training, conditioning and restructuring. Hypnotic imagery can be used for (a) systematic desensitization (using imagination the patient rehearses coping with *in vivo* difficult situations), (b) restructuring of cognitive processes at various levels of awareness or consciousness, (c) exploration of the remote past (regression work), and (d) directing attention to positive experiences.

Dream induction

Hypnosis can be utilized to induce dreams and increase dream recall and understanding (Golden *et al.*, 1987). Hypnotic dream induction thus provides another vehicle for uncovering unconscious maladaptive thoughts, fantasies, feelings and images.

Expansion of experience across time

In addition to facilitating diverse emotional experience, hypnosis also provides a vehicle for exploring and expanding experience in the present, the past and the future. Such strategies can enhance divergent thinking and facilitate the reconstruction of dysfunctional 'realities'.

Mood induction

Negative or positive moods can be easily induced and modulated by hypnosis, which makes it a useful method for teaching patients (through rehearsal) strategies for modulating and controlling negative or inappropriate affects. Hypnotic mood induction can also facilitate recall. Bower (1981) has provided evidence that certain materials can only be recalled when experiencing the coincident mood (mood-state-dependent memory).

Post-hypnotic suggestions

Post-hypnotic suggestions, especially when delivered during deep trance, can be very powerful in altering problem behaviors, dysfunctional cognitions and negative emotions. Post-hypnotic suggestions can also be used to shape efficacious behavior. Barrios (1973) considers post-hypnotic suggestion to be a form of 'higher-order-conditioning', which can function as positive or negative reinforcement for increasing or decreasing the probability of desired or undesired behaviors, respectively. Drawing on this idea, Clarke and Jackson (1983) have utilized post-hypnotic suggestions to enhance the effect of *in vivo* exposure among agoraphobics.

Positive self-hypnosis

The focus of modern hypnotherapy is on empowering patients by teaching them self-help skills, such as self-hypnosis training, that can be easily transferred to real situations. Self-hypnotic skills increase confidence and reduce dependence on the therapist. Self-hypnosis training can be enhanced by hetero-hypnotic* induction and post-hypnotic suggestions. Most of the techniques mentioned above can be practiced under self-hypnosis, thus fostering positive self-hypnosis by deflecting preoccupation away from negative self-suggestions.

Perception of self-efficacy

Positive hypnotic experience, coupled with the belief that one has the ability to utilize self-hypnosis to alter symptoms, gives one an expectancy of self-efficacy, which can enhance treatment outcome. According to Bandura (1977), expectation of self-efficacy is central to all forms of therapeutic change.

---

* In the clinical setting it is advisable to start with hetero-hypnosis (hypnosis induced by the therapist) and then introduce the concept of self-hypnosis, as this increases the patient's confidence in self-hypnosis.

Easy integration

Hypnotherapy provides a broad range of short-term techniques, which can be easily integrated with many forms of therapy (e.g. with behavior therapy, cognitive therapy, developmental therapy, psychodynamic therapy, supportive therapy). Because hypnosis itself is not a therapy, the specific treatment effects will be contingent on the therapeutic approach with which it is integrated. Nevertheless, the hypnotic relationship can enhance the efficacy of therapy when hypnosis is used as an adjunct to a particular form of therapy (Brown and Fromm, 1986).

Limitations of hypnosis

Lacks unique theoretical underpinnings

As mentioned before, hypnotherapy is a set of short-term clinical techniques. Hypnosis itself does not provide a theory of personality or psychopathology. A theoretical framework for conceptualizing hypnotic treatment is therefore lacking, and the manner in which hypnotherapy produces therapeutic outcomes is very often unclear. Hypnotherapy, as a rule, tends to be used in a shotgun fashion without giving adequate attention to the disorder being treated and without stating how hypnotherapy *per se* will be used to alleviate the symptoms (Wadden and Anderton, 1982).

Over-emphasis on unconscious factors

Influenced by the works of Charcot, Freud and Janet, hypnotherapy was long dominated by psychodynamic theories of psychopathology, and therapists tended to over-emphasize the importance of unconscious factors in the causation of psychological and psychosomatic disorders. This resulted in a propensity to underplay the role of conscious cognitions (e.g. attitudes, beliefs, fantasies, self-talk and thinking), overt behaviors and environmental factors, which can also cause and maintain symptoms and maladaptive behaviors. In fact, conscious and symptomatic interventions were considered harmful within the framework of psychodynamic psychotherapy.

For example, some well-known and respected hypnotherapists such as Brenman and Gill (1947) and Fromm (1984) argued that permanent change will not occur unless the patient's unconscious conflicts are uncovered and worked through. Although these approaches may be helpful to some patients, they have hindered the expansion and exploration of other models of etiology and intervention. This has resulted in hypnotherapy making little progress or impact with certain disorders (e.g. depression, obsessive-compulsive disorder). Moreover, these attitudes created the myth that hypnosis is harmful with certain psychological disorders, such as depression (Hartland, 1971). Alladin (1989, 1994, 2006, 2007; Alladin and Heap, 1991) and Yapko (1992, 2001) have challenged these beliefs and have demonstrated that when hypnotherapy is appropriately combined with cognitive therapy, it can become a very effective treatment for clinical depression.

Passivity in therapy

In line with the traditional omnipotent and omniscient view of psychoanalysts, the patient has taken a passive role in hypnotherapy. The patient is not informed how the hypnotherapy will help him or her, or modify the underlying pathology. Often patients are offered post-hypnotic suggestions, but as a rule they are not actively involved in monitoring and restructuring thoughts, feelings, behaviors and physiological responses. In fact, active participation from the patient should be encouraged, especially when treating such chronic psychological disorders as anxiety, depression or chronic pain.

Hypnosis is not therapy

Hypnotic induction, on its own, has no therapeutic value. Hypnotic techniques are mainly used as adjuncts to other forms of psychotherapy. Unfortunately this integration can cause confusion. At times it is difficult to differentiate hypnotic adjunctive techniques from other cognitive behavioral interventions, although some hypnotherapists insist on calling the adjunctive techniques hypnotherapy. However, Wadden and Anderton (1982) state that 'it is unclear from both a theoretical and practical standpoint what criteria are used to identify a treatment as uniquely hypnotic'. Instead of defining a treatment as hypnotherapy just by labelling it as such (Lazarus, 1973), it would be more beneficial to examine the similarities and differences between the hypnotic and non-hypnotic treatment procedures and try to ensure they complement each other to increase the treatment effect.

Symptom removal

To a large extent hypnotherapy focuses on symptom removal. Few attempts are made to teach and establish active coping skills. Even Ericksonian therapists, who talk of unconscious experiential learning, do not directly teach coping skills to their patients; instead they focus on symptom relief. In fact, some of these therapists believe direct intervention produces patient resistance. Moreover, traditionally hypnotherapists have not actively addressed maladaptive cognitions and behaviors. In such chronic conditions as anxiety and depression, 'insight-oriented methods based on persuasion, reasoning and re-education are necessary to achieve symptom alleviation' (Golden *et al.*, 1987, pp. 1–2) and 'therapeutic results are more enduring if symptom amelioration includes the modification of thoughts, feelings, and behavior patterns that maintain the symptoms' (Golden *et al.*, 1987, p. 7).

Negative self-hypnosis not addressed

Although hypnotherapists usually emphasize teaching their patients self-hypnosis, the influence of negative self-hypnosis (NSH) (Araoz, 1981, 1985) is not actively addressed. Routine self-hypnosis unmindful of the power of NSH can be easily countered by NSH, thus minimizing treatment effect. When teaching self-hypnosis, both patient and therapist should be aware of the powerful sabotaging effect of NSH.

Hypotheses lack support

Data are rarely provided to support the hypotheses as to why hypnotherapy works. For instance, the efficacy of hypnosis is often attributed to either heightened expectancy (Lazarus, 1973), the therapeutic effects of the trance state (Weitzenhoffer, 1963), or enhancement of bodily relaxation and visual imagery (Kroger and Fezler, 1976), but the data are rarely provided to support them.

DEFINITION OF HYPNOSIS AND TRANCE

Recently, the Division of Psychological Hypnosis (Division 30) of the American Psychological Association (Green *et al.*, 2005) defined and described hypnosis as a procedure during which the subject is told that suggestions for imaginative experiences will be presented. The hypnotic induction is an extended initial suggestion for one's imagination, and may contain further elaborations of introduction. A hypnotic procedure is used to encourage and evaluate responses to suggestions.

When using hypnosis, one person (the subject) is guided by another (the hypnotist) to respond to suggestions for changes in subjective experience, alterations in perception, sensation, emotion, thought or behavior. People can also learn self-hypnosis, which is the act of administering hypnotic procedures on oneself. If the subject responds to hypnotic suggestions, it is generally inferred that hypnosis has been induced. Many believe that hypnotic responses and experiences are characteristic of a hypnotic state. While some think that it is not necessary to use the word 'hypnosis' as part of the hypnotic induction, others view it as essential.

The Division 30 definition of hypnosis also focused on the issues of hypnotic procedures, relaxation and hypnotic responsivity (Green *et al.*, 2005). Details of hypnotic procedures and suggestions will differ depending on the goals of the practitioner and purposes of the clinical or research endeavor. Procedures traditionally involve suggestions to relax, although relaxation is not necessary for hypnosis, and a wide variety of suggestions can be used, including those to become more alert.

Suggestions that permit the extent of hypnosis to be assessed by comparing responses to standardized scales can be used in both clinical and research settings. Although the majority of individuals are responsive to at least some suggestions, scores on standardized scales range from high to negligible. Traditionally, scores are grouped into low, medium and high. As is the case with other positively scaled measures of psychological constructs, such as attention and awareness, the salience of evidence for having achieved hypnosis increases with an individual's score.

The British definition of hypnosis is less descriptive than the APA Division 30 definition and the focus is more on the interaction between the hypnotist and the subject. For instance, Heap and Aravind (2002, p. 55), in the well-known text *Hartland's Medical and Dental Hypnosis*, state:

> The term 'hypnosis' is used to denote an interaction between two people (or one person and a group) in which one of them, the hypnotist, by means of verbal communication, encourages the other, the subject or subjects, to focus their attention away from their immediate realities and concerns and on inner experiences such as thoughts, feelings and imagery. The hypnotist further attempts to create alterations in the subject's sensations, perceptions, feelings, thoughts and behaviour by directing them to imagine various events or situations that, were they to occur in reality, would evoke the intended changes.

Given that hypnosis is a multidimensional experience and there are many theories of hypnosis, the definition is laudable in its attempt to consolidate the different views of hypnosis while trying to counter public misconceptions. However, the definition has been criticized for being too broad and too descriptive (e.g. Nash, 2005; Yapko, 2003). This is not surprising because hypnosis practitioners and researchers hold different theoretical viewpoints. The APA

Division 30 committee (Green *et al.*, 2005, p. 262) is aware of this limitation and recommends further refining the definition:

> 'The current definition and description need not be considered a finished product. Hopefully, it will continue to evolve as various hypnosis organizations grapple with it and as new data add to our understanding of hypnosis' (1994b, p. 162). We strongly agree with these sentiments. We echo the call for future committees and groups to evaluate research that makes it possible to critique, update, and ultimately challenge the . . . definition. The intent is to welcome improvement to our science as well as informing the public about hypnosis.

Definition of hypnotic trance

Zarren and Eimer (2002, p. 4) describe the hypnotic trance as an altered state that is produced by a formal hypnotic induction ritual or ceremony that serves as the focusing method. In contrast to hypnotic trances that are formally induced for therapeutic purposes, there are informal trances that occur spontaneously without any formal hypnotic induction ceremony. Zarren and Eimer (2002, p. 4) differentiate between hypnosis state and trance state:

> In the clinical setting, a hypnosis state, as differentiated from a trance state, can be induced without a formal trance induction. This occurs when a clinician communicates with a patient in language and form that are acceptable to the patient's conscious and unconscious minds. We term this form of communication waking state reframing. In our view, the subsequent formal induction of hypnotic trance serves to fix the information communicated further in place in the patient's unconscious.

Humphreys (2000) has listed 20 overlapping basic characteristics of the hypnotic trance as an altered state of consciousness (summarized by Zarren and Eimer, 2002, pp. 6–7):

○ narrowed focus of attention

○ increased absorption and reduced distractibility

○ inattention to or disinterest in environmental stimuli other than the therapist

○ increased concentration on a particular aspect of experience (e.g. sensation)

- ○ increased suggestibility
- ○ reduction of critical evaluation and screening
- ○ reduction of voluntary activity (mental and/or physical)
- ○ passive responsiveness or non-volitional activity
- ○ relative effortlessness
- ○ reduction in internal dialogue or self-talk
- ○ alteration of cognitive functions
- ○ facilitation of atypical modes of thinking, such as 'trance logic'
- ○ heightened rapport with the therapist
- ○ some degree of physical relaxation or comfort
- ○ altered sense of one's body
- ○ increased imaginal processing
- ○ time distortion
- ○ alteration of memory processing
- ○ relative dominance of the parasympathetic branch
- ○ relative dominance of right hemispheric cerebral functioning.

A working definition of hypnosis

As mentioned earlier, this book adopts a state (neodissociation) theory of hypnosis which is widely used in the clinical domain. Within this context I find the following definition and description of hypnosis proposed by Maldonado and Spiegel useful (2003, p. 1285):

> Hypnosis is a natural state of aroused, attentive focal concentration coupled with relative suspension of peripheral awareness. It involves an intensity of focus that allows the hypnotized person to make maximal use of innate abilities to control perception, memory, and somatic function. Hypnotic capacities represents both a potential vulnerability to certain kinds of psychiatric illness, such as post-traumatic stress, conversion, and dissociative disorders, and an asset, in that it can facilitate various psychotherapeutic strategies. Because hypnotic capacity is a normal and widely distributed trait, and because entry into hypnotic states occurs spontaneously, hypnotic phenomena occur frequently. Even psychiatrists who make no formal use of hypnosis can enhance their effectiveness by learning to recognize and take advantage of hypnotic mental states.

REFERENCES

Alladin A. (1989). Cognitive-hypnotherapy for depression. In: Waxman D, Pederson D, Wilkie I, *et al.*, editors. *Hypnosis: the 4th European Congress at Oxford* (pp. 175–82). London: Whurr Publishers.

Alladin A. (1994). Cognitive hypnotherapy with depression. *Journal of Cognitive Psychotherapy: An International Quarterly* 8(4): 275–88.

Alladin A. (2006). Cognitive hypnotherapy for treating depression. In: Chapman R, editor. *The Clinical Use of Hypnosis in Cognitive Behavior Therapy: a practitioner's casebook* (pp. 139–87). New York: Springer Publishing Company.

Alladin A. (2007). *Handbook of Cognitive Hypnotherapy for Depression: an evidence-based approach.* Philadelphia: Lippincott Williams and Wilkins.

Alladin A, Heap M. (1991). Hypnosis and depression. In: Heap M, Dryden W, editors. *Hypnotherapy: a handbook* (pp. 49–67). Milton Keynes: Open University Press.

Araoz DL. (1981). Negative self-hypnosis. *Journal of Contemporary Psychotherapy* 12: 45–52.

Araoz DL. (1985). *The New Hypnosis.* New York: Brunner/Mazel Publishers.

Bandura A. (1977). Self-efficacy: toward a unifying theory of behavioural change. *Psychological Review* 84: 191–215.

Barber TX. (1969). *Hypnosis: a scientific approach.* New York: Van Nostrand Reinhold.

Barber TX. (1979). Suggested ('hypnotic') behavior: the trance paradigm versus an alternative paradigm. In: Fromm E, Shor RE, editors. *Hypnosis: developments in research and new perspectives.* 2nd ed. New York: Aldine.

Barber TX. (1984). Changing 'unchangeable' bodily processes by (hypnotic) suggestions: a new look at hypnosis, cognitions, imagining, and the mind-body problem: In: Sheikh AA, editor. *Imagination and Healing* (pp. 69–127). Farmingdale, NY: Baywood.

Barber TX. (1999). A comprehensive three-dimensional theory of hypnosis. In: Kirsch I, Capafons A, Cardena-Buelna E, *et al.*, editors. *Clinical Hypnosis and Self-Regulation: cognitive-behavioral perspective* (pp. 21–48). Washington, DC: American Psychological Association.

Barrios AA. (1973). Posthypnotic suggestion in high-order conditioning: a methodological and experimental analysis. *International Journal of Clinical and Experimental Hypnosis* 21: 32–50.

Boutin G. (1978). The treatment of test anxiety by rational stage directed hypnotherapy. *American Journal of Clinical Hypnosis* 21: 52.

Bower GH. (1981). Mood and memory. *American Psychologist* 36: 129–48.

Brenman M, Gill MM. (1947). *Hypnotherapy: a survey of the literature.* Oxford: International Universities Press.

Brown PD, Fromm E. (1986). *Hypnotherapy and Hypnoanalysis.* Hillsdale, NJ: Erlbaum.

Clarke JC, Jackson JA. (1983). *Hypnosis and Behavior Therapy: the treatment of anxiety and phobias.* New York: Springer.

Dengrove E. (1973). The use of hypnosis in behaviour therapy. *International Journal of Clinical and Experimental Hypnosis* 21: 13–17.

De Piano FA, Salzberg HC. (1981). Hypnosis as an aid to recall of meaningful information presented under three types of arousal. *International Journal of Clinical and Experimental Hypnosis* 29: 283–400.

Erickson MH, Rossi E. (1979). *Hypnotherapy: an exploratory casebook.* New York: Irvington.

Feldman JB. (2004). The neurobiology of pain, affect and hypnosis. *American Journal of Clinical Hypnosis* 46: 187–200.

Freiderich M, Trippe R, Ozcan M, *et al.* (2001). Laser-evoked potentials to noxious stimulation during hypnotic analgesia and distraction of attention suggest different brain mechanisms of pain control. *Psychophysiology* 38: 768–76.

Fromm E. (1977). An ego-psychological theory for altered states of consciousness. *International Journal of Clinical and Experimental Psychology* 25: 373–87.

Fromm E. (1984). Theory and practice of hypnoanalysis. In: Wester WC, Smith A, editors. *Clinical Hypnosis: a multidisciplinary approach* (pp. 142–54). New York: Lippincott.

Furster JM. (1995). *Memory in the Cerebral Cortex.* Boston: MIT Press.

Gazzaniga M, editor. (2000). *The New Cognitive Neurosciences.* Cambridge, MA: MIT Press.

Gill MM, Brenman M. (1959). *Hypnosis and Related States: psychoanalytic studies in regression.* New York: International Universities Press.

Golden WL, Dowd ET, Friedberg F. (1987). *Hypnotherapy: a modern approach.* New York: Pergamon Press.

Green JP, Barabasz A, Barrett D, *et al.* (2005). Forging ahead: the 2003 APA Division 30 definition of hypnosis. *Journal of Clinical and Experimental Hypnosis* 53: 259–64.

Gruzelier J. (1998). A working model of the neurophysiology of hypnosis: a review of the evidence. *Contemporary Hypnosis* 15: 3–21.

Gruzelier J. (2005). Altered states of consciousness and hypnosis in the twenty-first century. *Contemporary Hypnosis* 22: 1–7.

Hartland, J. (1971). *Medical and Dental Hypnosis and its Clinical Applications.* 2nd ed. London: Bailliere Tindall.

Heap M, editor. (1988). *Hypnosis: current clinical, experimental and forensic practices.* London: Croom Helm.

Heap M, Aravind KK. (2002). *Hartland's Medical and Dental Hypnosis.* 4th ed. London: Churchill Livingstone.

Hilgard ER. (1973). The domain of hypnosis: with some comments on alternate paradigms. *American Psychologist* 28: 972–82.

Hilgard ER. (1974). Toward a neo-dissociation theory: multiple cognitive controls in human functioning. *Perspectives in Biology and Medicine* 17: 301–16.

Hilgard ER. (1986). *Divided Consciousness: multiple controls in human thought and action.* New York: John Wiley and Sons.

Hilgard ER. (1991). A neodissociation interpretation of hypnosis. In: Lynn SJ, Rhue JW, editors. *Theories of Hypnosis: current models and perspectives* (pp. 83–104). New York: Guilford Press.

Humphreys RB. (2000). *The Neurobiology of Hypnosis.* Advanced workshop presented at the annual meeting of the American Society of Clinical Hypnosis, Baltimore.

Janet P. (1889). *L'Automatisme psychologique.* Paris: Felix Alcan.

Janet. P. (1907). *The Major Symptoms of Hysteria.* New York: Macmillan.

Kallio S, Revonsuo A. (2003). Hypnotic phenomena and altered states of consciousness: a multilevel framework of description and explanation. *Contemporary Hypnosis* 20: 111–64.

Kihlstrom JF. (2003). The fox, the hedgehog, and hypnosis. *International Journal of Clinical and Experimental Hypnosis* 51: 166–89.

Kihlstrom JF, Barnier AJ. (2005). The hidden observer: a straw horse, undeservedly flogged. *Contemporary Hypnosis* 22: 144–51.

Kirsch I. (2000). The response set theory of hypnosis. *American Journal of Clinical Hypnosis* 42(3–4): 274–93.

Kirsch I. (2005). Empirical resolution of the altered state debate. *Contemporary Hypnosis* 22: 18–23.

Kohut H. (1977). *The Restoration of the Self.* New York: International Universities.

Kosslyn SM, Thompson WL, Costantini-Ferrando MF, *et al.* (2000). Hypnotic visual illusion alters color processing in the brain. *American Journal of Psychiatry* 157: 1279–84.

Kroger WS, Fezler WD. (1976). *Hypnosis and Behavior Modification: imagery conditioning.* Philadelphia: JB Lippincott Company.

Lazarus AA. (1973). 'Hypnosis' as a facilitator in behavior therapy. *International Journal of Clinical and Experimental Hypnosis* 6: 83–9.

Ley RG, Freeman RJ. (1984). Imagery, cerebral laterality, and the healing process. In: Sheikh AA, editor. *Imagination and Healing* (pp. 51–68). New York: Baywood Publishing Co. Inc.

Llinas RR, Pare D. (1991). Of dreaming and wakefulness. *Neuroscience* 44: 521–35.

Ludwig AM. (1966). Altered states of consciousness. In: Tart CT, editor. *Altered States of Consciousness* (pp. 9–22). New York: John Wiley and Sons.

Lynn SJ, Kirsch I. (2006). *Essentials of Clinical Hypnosis: an evidence-based approach.* Washington, DC: American Psychological Association.

Maldonado JR, Spiegel D. (2003). Hypnosis. In: Hales RE, Yudofsky SC, editors. *Textbook of Clinical Psychiatry.* 4th ed. (pp. 1285–331). Washington, D.C.: American Psychiatric Publishing.

Mesulam MM, editor. (2000). *Principles of Behavioural and Cognitive Neurology*. Oxford: Oxford University Press.

Nadon R, Laurence JR, Perry C. (1991). The two disciplines of scientific hypnosis: a synergistic model: In: Lynn SJ, Rhue JW, editors. *Theories of Hypnosis: current models and perspectives* (pp. 485–519). New York: Guilford Press.

Naish P. (2005). Detecting hypnotically altered states of consciousness. *Contemporary Hypnosis* 22: 24–30.

Nash MR. (2005). The importance of being earnest when crafting definitions. *International Journal of Clinical and Experimental Hypnosis* 53: 265–80.

Orne MT. (1959). The nature of hypnosis: artifact and essence. *Journal of Abnormal Psychology* 58: 277–99.

Rainville P, Hofbauer RK, Bushnell MC, *et al.* (2002). Hypnosis modulates activity in brain structures involved in the regulation of consciousness. *Journal of Cognitive Neuroscience* 14: 887–901.

Rowley DT. (1986). *Hypnosis and Hypnotherapy*. London: Croom Helm.

Shor RE. (1959). Hypnosis and the concept of the generalized reality-orientation. *American Journal of Psychotherapy* 13: 582–602.

Spanos NP, Barber TX. (1974). Toward a convergence in hypnosis research. *American Psychologist* 29: 500–11.

Spanos NP, Coe WC. (1992). A social psychological approach to hypnosis. In: Fromm E, Nash MR, editors. *Contemporary Hypnosis Research* (pp. 102–30). New York: Guilford Press.

Spanos NP, Hewitt EC. (1980). The hidden observer in hypnotic analgesia: discovery or experimental creation? *Journal of Personality and Social Psychology* 39: 1201–14.

Spanos NP, Radtke HL, Bertrand LD. (1984). Hypnotic amnesia as a strategic enactment: breaching amnesia in highly hypnotizable subjects. *Journal of Personality and Social Psychology* 47: 1155–69.

Spiegel D. (2005). Multileveling the playing field: altering our state of consciousness to understand hypnosis. *Contemporary Hypnosis* 22: 31–3.

Szechtman H, Woody E, Bowers KS, *et al.* (1998). Where the imaginal appears real: a positron emission tomography study of auditory hallucinations. *Proceedings of the National Academy of Sciences* 95: 1956–60.

Tart C. (1975). *States of Consciousness*. New York: Dutton.

Tosi DJ, Baisden BS. (1984). Cognitive-experiential therapy and hypnosis. In: Wester WC, Smith AH, editors. *Clinical Hypnosis: a multidisciplinary approach* (pp. 155–78). New York: JB Lippincott.

Vaitl D, Birbaumer N, Gruzelier J, *et al.* (2005). Psychobiology of altered states of consciousness. *Psychology Bulletin* 131: 98–127.

Wadden TA, Anderton CH. (1982). The clinical use of hypnosis. *Psychological Bulletin* 91: 215–43.

Watkins JG, Watkins HH. (1979). Ego states and hidden observers. *Journal of Altered States of Consciousness* 5: 3–18.

Weitzenhoffer AM. (1963). *Hypnotism: an objective study in suggestibility*. New York: John Wiley and Sons.

West LJ. (1967). Dissociative reaction. In: Freedman AM, Kaplan HI, editors. *Comprehensive Textbook of Psychiatry*. Baltimore: Williams and Wilkins Co.

Woody E, Sadler P. (1998). On reintegrating dissociated theories: comment on Kirsch and Lynn (1998). *Psychological Bulletin* 123: 192–7.

Yapko MD. (1992). *Hypnosis and the Treatment of Depressions: strategies for change*. New York: Brunner/Mazel.

Yapko MD. (2001). *Treating Depression with Hypnosis: integrating cognitive-behavioral and strategic approaches*. New York: Brunner/Routledge.

Yapko MD. (2003). *Trancework: an introduction to the practice of clinical hypnosis*. 3rd ed. New York: Brunner-Routledge.

Zarren JI, Eimer BN. (2002). *Brief Cognitive Hypnosis: facilitating the change of dysfunctional behavior*. New York: Springer Publishing Company.

Zeman A. (2001). Consciousness. *Brain* 124: 1263–89.

CHAPTER 2

Stages of Hypnotherapy

SUMMARY

This chapter describes eight sequential stages of hypnotherapy: preparing the patient for hypnosis, hypnotic induction, deepening of hypnosis, therapeutic utilization of hypnosis, ego-strengthening, post-hypnotic suggestions, self-hypnosis, and termination of hypnosis. With experience, the therapist will be able to choose the sequence of treatment according to the clinical needs of the individual patient. The chapter also provides a contemporary framework for conducting clinical assessment within the context of case formulation. Such an approach to treatment becomes principle-driven, rather than delivering treatment in a hit-and-miss fashion. The chapter also provides a full script for hypnotic induction, deepening and ego-strengthening, which can easily be adapted to the needs of a variety of patients.

INTRODUCTION

Hypnotherapy can be subdivided into eight stages: preparing the patient for hypnosis, hypnotic induction, deepening of hypnosis, therapeutic utilization of hypnosis, ego-strengthening, post-hypnotic suggestions, self-hypnosis and termination of hypnosis. The purpose of this chapter is to describe these eight stages of hypnotherapy.

STAGE 1: PREPARING THE PATIENT FOR HYPNOSIS

Successful hypnotic induction and hypnotherapy require satisfactory preparation of the patient. Good preparation involves information gathering (clinical assessment), establishing rapport, assessing for hypnotic suggestibility, clarifying misconceptions about hypnosis, providing facilitating information, and organizing the setting for hypnotherapy.

Information gathering

Before initiating hypnotherapy, it is important for the therapist to take a detailed clinical history and identify the essential psychological, physiological and social aspects of the patient's behaviors. This should include functional and dysfunctional patterns of thinking, feeling, bodily responses and behaviors. To make a reliable diagnosis, the therapist is advised to use standard diagnostic criteria such as the *Diagnostic and Statistical Manual of Mental Disorders* (4th ed.) (American Psychiatric Association, 2000), or the International Classification of Diseases (ICD-10) (World Health Organization, 1992). Specific psychometric measures such as the Beck Depression Inventory – Revised (Beck *et al.*, 1996), the Beck Anxiety Inventory (Beck and Steer, 1993a), the Beck Hopelessness Scale (Beck and Steer, 1993b), and the Revised Hamilton Rating Scale for Depression (RHRSD, Warren,1994) can also be administered to determine the severity of the symptoms before, during and after treatment.

Currently there is a strong movement for conducting clinical assessment within the context of *case formulation*. The main function of a case formulation is to devise an effective treatment plan. Evidence suggests that matching treatment to particular patient characteristics improves outcome (Beutler *et al.*, 2000). By conceptualizing a case, the clinician develops a working hypothesis on how the patient's problems can be understood in terms of a theoretical framework. This provides a compass or a guide to understanding the treatment process.

Needleman (2003) views case formulation as the process of developing an explicit parsimonious understanding of the patients and their problems that effectively guides treatment. Within this framework, treatment begins with an assessment, which generates a hypothesis about the mechanisms causing or maintaining the symptoms. The hypothesis is the individualized case formulation, which the therapist uses to develop an individualized treatment plan. As treatment proceeds, the therapist collects data via further assessment to evaluate the effects of the planned treatment.

If it becomes evident that the treatment is not working, the therapist reformulates the case and develops a new treatment plan, which is also monitored and evaluated. Clinical work thus becomes more systematic and hypothesis-driven. Such an approach to treatment becomes principle-driven rather than delivering treatment strategies randomly or in a predetermined order.

In order to identify the mechanisms that underlie the patient's problem within the context of hypnotherapy, I use an eight-step case formulation (*see* Alladin, 2007), derived from the work of Persons *et al.* (2001) and Ledley *et al.*, 2005). The eight components, summarized in Table 2.1, are described in detail below. Appendix 2A supplies a template for cognitive hypnotherapy case formulation and a treatment plan, and Appendix 2B provides the formulated case and treatment plan for Cathy, a 32-year-old divorced woman with a 10-year history of recurrent major depressive disorder. Chapter 5 provides a comprehensive approach, 'Hypnotherapy with a Psychiatric Disorder: Depression', for treating clinical depression. This hypnotherapy approach combines hypnosis and cognitive behavior therapy in the management of chronic depression.

TABLE 2.1 Eight-step case formulation

---

1. List the major symptoms and problems in functioning.
2. Formulate a formal psychiatric diagnosis.
3. Formulate a working hypothesis.
4. Identify the precipitants and activating situations.
5. Explore the origin of negative self-schemas (deeper beliefs).
6. Summarize the working hypothesis.
7. Outline the treatment plan.
8. Identify strengths and assets and predict obstacles to treatment.

Establishing rapport

Establishing rapport with the patient is of vital importance. Without good rapport the patient may not allow himself or herself to fully experience the hypnotic trance. Modern hypnotherapy is a collaborative venture, involving co-operation from both the patient and the therapist. Araoz (1981, 1985) has described the TEAM approach for the development of *trust* and positive *expectations* and *attitudes*, and for the utilization of the patient's *motivation* in hypnotherapy. Golden *et al.* (1987) define rapport as the development of this TEAM approach, which can be established within the hypnotherapy context by:

- ❍ the therapist showing warmth, empathy and caring

- ❍ developing trust by utilizing the therapist's prestige, expertise and authority

- ❍ the therapist demonstrating good understanding of the patient's problems

- ❍ the therapist 'joining' the patient; that is, being able to speak the patient's 'language'

- ❍ tailoring treatment to the expectations of the patient.

Assessing hypnotic suggestibility

Some clinicians prefer to assess their patient for hypnotic suggestibility in order to determine whether the patient will benefit from hypnotherapy. These clinicians take the view that hypnotic suggestibility is a stable trait that cannot be significantly modified by training. Other clinicians disagree. My own view, based on 25 years of clinical experience, is that some individuals are more talented than others at experiencing hypnosis. I agree with Barabasz and Watkin's (2005, p. 89) position that hypnosis is not 'a special process with a one-dimensional EEG brain signature' or an 'either-or' state, but a multidimensional experience reflecting 'various subjective states perceived by the participant'. However, this multidimensional experience is 'a matter of degree' (Barabasz and Watkins, 2005, p. 89).

Some individuals can easily enter into a deep trance state and experience full-blown regression, time distortion, significant somatosensory changes and vivid hallucinations. Others may feel relaxed or carry out simple suggestions but are unable to experience major changes in their body or perceptions. I prefer testing for hypnotic suggestibility for several clinical reasons.

- ❍ A standardized suggestibility test provides an indication of the degree of hypnotic depth the patient can experience. This information is important in selecting treatment strategies. Some hypnotherapeutic techniques (e.g. full-blown regression, anesthesia) require a deep state of hypnosis, while others (e.g. moderate relaxation) require a light hypnotic state.

○ The test helps the patient become familiar with hypnotic-like experience prior to hypnotic induction. Such experience helps debunk the myths surrounding hypnosis and prepares the patient for hypnotic induction.

○ It alleviates fears and so helps to build rapport and trust.

○ The administration of the test creates a positive psychological set and so makes later induction of deep hypnosis easier.

○ From the test the therapist can assess the patient's response to suggestions (e.g. feeling light or heavy), which can be integrated into future sessions of hypnotherapy.

Clarifying the misconceptions about hypnosis

Yapko (2003) has listed 14 misconceptions about hypnosis. After establishing rapport with the patient, it is important to educate and reassure the patient about these misconceptions.

○ *Hypnosis is a good thing:* hypnosis is not inherently good. Hypnosis itself does not cure people. It has the potential to be utilized as a powerful tool for reducing suffering and promoting healing.

○ *Hypnosis is effected by the power of the hypnotist:* as noted earlier, hypno-therapy is a collaborative venture between the hypnotist and the therapist. Without the patient's co-operation, hypnosis cannot take place.

○ *Only certain types of people can be hypnotized:* although there is controversy as to whether some people are hypnotizable or not, it is generally accepted that hypnotic responsiveness in people along a continuum, ranging from low hypnotizables to very high hypnotizables. Therefore, individuals cannot all experience the same deep trance level.

○ *Anyone who is hypnotized is weak-minded:* this misconception is based on the all-powerful Svengali image of the hypnotist portrayed in novels and movies. The ability to be hypnotized is not correlated with any specific personality defect or negative trait. Moreover, each person has a capacity for will and virtually all people have the ability to enter spontaneous or informal hypnotic states regularly.

○ *Once one has been hypnotized, one can no longer resist it:* this misconception is based on the idea that a hypnotist controls the will of his or her subject and once one succumbs to the power of the hypnotist, one is forever at his or her mercy. Since the hypnotic process is an interaction between the patient and the hypnotist, based on mutual power and trust to attain a certain desirable therapeutic outcome, the patient may choose to experience, or not, the hypnotic trance.

○ *One can be hypnotized to say or do something against one's will:* it is true that brainwashing and other untoward influences have been used. In the clinical context, however, the relationship between the clinician and the patient is one of mutual responsibility and accountability. In theory the clinician provides benevolent suggestions that the patient can either accept or reject. It is also worth noting that the conditions necessary to effect brainwashing 'are not in and of themselves hypnosis' (Yapko, 1995).

○ *Being hypnotized can be hazardous:* hypnosis in itself is not harmful. If any harm occurs, it is usually due to the incompetence of the therapist, who may be ignorant about the complexity of the patient's mind, or ignorant about the condition being treated, or lack respect for others.

○ *One becomes dependent on the hypnotist:* hypnosis as a therapeutic tool in itself does not foster dependence on the therapist. Although some dependence in the initial stages of hypnosis may be desirable (to provide help and comfort and to build trust and therapeutic alliance), a good clinician knows that the ultimate goal of responsible therapy is to help the patient establish self-reliance and independence.

○ *One can become stuck in hypnosis:* since hypnosis is a state of focused attention, controlled by the patient, the patient can decide to terminate the experience at any time.

○ *One is asleep or unconscious when in hypnosis:* although the patient may experience generalized relaxation when in a trance state, the person is not asleep or unconscious. The hypnotized person, irrespective of the depth of trance state, has some level of awareness.

○ *Hypnosis is therapy:* hypnosis is not a therapy. It is a therapeutic tool that is used as an adjunct to other forms of therapy (medical or psychological). When hypnosis is used as adjunctive intervention, it is referred to as *clinical hypnosis* or *hypnotherapy*. Despite its name, hypnotherapy itself is not a therapy as hypnotherapy does not belong to any specific school of therapy. It is used as an adjunct to enhance treatment effect.

○ *One must be relaxed to experience hypnosis:* since hypnosis is a state of concentrated attention, physical relaxation is not a prerequisite for hypnosis to occur. A person can be hypnotized while involved in physical activities such as riding an exercise bike.

○ *Hypnosis produces accurate recall of everything that happened to one:* the mind does not work like a computer, taking in and storing the exact experience so that it can be accurately recalled later. Memory is a dynamic constructive process and therefore memory can be unreliable. Hypnosis does not facilitate recall of accurate memory.

Providing facilitative information

After debunking the myths and misconceptions of hypnosis, it is advisable to provide your patient with 'facilitative information' about hypnotherapy (Lynn and Kirsch, 2006, p. 45). According to Lynn and Kirsch, such facilitative information elicits the patient's active co-operation and makes it easier for the patient to experience suggested effects. Some of the facilitative information provided by Lynn and Kirsch (2006, pp. 45–6) includes the following.

○ Hypnosis is something that a patient does or participates in; it is not something done to the patient. Therefore the patient's co-operation is very important.

○ Hypnotic suggestions are experienced more vividly when a person actively imagines their occurrence. For example, suggested arm levitation can be experienced more easily if the participant intentionally imagines the arm is becoming lighter.

○ The hypnotic experience depends on the patient's beliefs and expectations.

Organizing the setting for hypnotherapy

It is recommended that hypnosis be conducted in a quiet room, although this may not always be possible. For example, a dentist practicing hypnosis in a busy office may not have the facility of a quiet setting. Although a quiet setting, gentle lighting and comfortable furniture are desirable, successful hypnotherapy can be conducted in all kinds of environments (Yapko, 2003) as long as the practitioner is not being interrupted constantly.

STAGE 2: HYPNOTIC INDUCTION

There are numerous procedures for inducing hypnosis. In this chapter I will focus on formal and standardized procedures that have been used with considerable success. These procedures provide the novice hypnotist with examples of hypnotic induction procedures which allow a comfortable start to practicing hypnosis. The procedures described here can be very effective with highly suggestible patients, and can be easily incorporated with other induction techniques.

The eye-fixation technique

The eye-fixation technique is perhaps the most popular form of hypnotic induction, especially among beginners. This is a very direct and simple approach to hypnosis. It involves having the subject fixate his or her gaze on some specific stimulus, which can be virtually anything: a spot on the wall or ceiling, a candle, a fireplace, etc. As the subject stares at the stimulus, the therapist encourages the subject to become aware of his or her eyes becoming relaxed and tired so that gradually the subject will want to close the eyes and drift into a very relaxed state. Here is a script for the eye-fixation technique, modified from Hartland (1971, p. 46).

THE EYE-FIXATION TECHNIQUE

Just make yourself comfortable in the chair and choose a spot on the ceiling and fixate your eyes on it. Do not turn your gaze anywhere else, just focus on the spot. Let yourself go limp and slack and let yourself relax as much as possible.

And gradually, you will begin to feel that your eyes are becoming tired, very tired. You feel your eyelids are feeling heavier and heavier. So heavy . . . that they feel they want to blink. As soon as they want to blink, just let them blink as much as they like. Let everything happen, just as it wants to happen. You feel your eyelids are beginning to blink already (*if the subject begins to blink, reinforce the suggestions*).

Very soon those blinks will become slower and bigger. And your eyelids will feel so very, very heavy and tired that they will want to close. Already, your eyes are becoming a bit watery and you are feeling very, very relaxed. Your eyelids feel so very, very heavy and tired that you want to let them close and drift into a very, very relaxed state.

You notice your eyes feel they want to close. Just let them go, they are closing now, closing, closing tighter and tighter. Just let yourself drift into a very deep, deep relaxed state.

The hand and arm levitation technique

The hand and arm levitation technique is another very popular method of hypnotic induction. Here is a standard script for hand and arm levitation technique for hypnotic induction.

THE HAND AND ARM LEVITATION TECHNIQUE

Just make yourself as comfortable as you can and rest your hands flat on your lap. Now, I would like you to look at your hands and become aware of the feelings and sensations in your fingers . . . As you become aware of the feelings and sensations in your fingers, sooner or later, you may notice a sensation, maybe in the tip of one of your fingers. This may happen, perhaps sooner than you expect . . . just wanting it to happen . . . and when it happens, you notice this experience and you may be wondering in which finger and in which hand this sensation is going to occur. When this happens, you will be really surprised that this is happening . . . and you can really enjoy noticing these important changes occurring.

Continue to enjoy noticing these changes occurring and soon you may notice these sensations changing into a movement so that the finger may, to your surprise, move upwards away from where it is resting right now (*comment on it and lightly and briefly touch the finger as soon as you notice this*) . . . and you will notice those sensations and movements gently flowing to the rest of your hand . . .

As these sensations and feelings spread over your hand, you begin to notice the whole hand and forearm becoming light, as light as a feather . . . As you notice your hand becoming lighter and lighter, you notice your hand begins to float effortlessly into the air, all by itself, floating all by itself, noticing that you do not need to do anything, your hand floating by itself . . . it is surprising how easy and relaxing this is . . . enjoying these important changes happening . . . As your hand floats toward your face, you feel you are becoming more and more relaxed and your eyes becoming heavier and heavier . . . and as soon as your hand touches your face you will close your eyes and drift into a very, very relaxed state.

Relaxation with counting method

Some practitioners prefer to combine hypnotic induction techniques; for example, the eye-fixation technique can be combined with the relaxation technique.

As many of my patients have anxiety, I find the combined relaxation with counting method very effective and beneficial to the patients. In Appendix 2C I have provided a complete script for the relaxation with counting method, together with the deepening technique and the ego-strengthening suggestions. Novice hypnotherapists may use the script verbatim initially, and then gradually adapt it to suit their own personal style and preference.

STAGE 3: DEEPENING OF HYPNOSIS

Once the trance has been initiated, it is useful to intensify the patient's involvement in the hypnotic experience and to capitalize on the patient's positive expectations for the hypnotic process. The intensification of the patient's involvement in the hypnotic experience is referred to as *trance deepening* (Braun and Horevitz, 1986). Hypnotic induction and deepening of trance are not distinct phases, but 'simply refer to the process of increasing the focus and concentration of attention by the patient' (Hammond, 1998, p. 71). Although it is not clear what we mean by deep hypnosis, most writers (e.g. Barabasz and Watkins, 2005; Golden *et al.*, 1987), from a clinical standpoint agree that 'most people experience hypnotic depth as increased feelings of relaxation, greater absorption or concentration and narrowing of one's attention, or, in the case of alert hypnosis, increased energy (Golden *et al.*, 1987).

In the clinical context, therefore, hypnotic trance is deepened to produce and demonstrate various hypnotic phenomena to the patient. Moreover, deepening of trance is a prerequisite to certain clinical strategies (e.g. a deep trance is required when a patient is undergoing surgery without chemical anesthesia, as noted by Barabasz and Watkins (2005, p. 185): 'varying levels of hypnotic depth [are] needed . . . to achieve a relaxation response . . . to achieve calmness . . . and let go in contrast to the level of depth essential for painless surgery without an anesthetic'.

The old concepts of stages or depth of hypnosis, based on the stages of sleep, are outdated now as hypnosis is no longer considered to be a state of sleep. Based on scientific knowledge, it is currently conceptualized that certain hypnotic phenomenon are more likely to occur when there are greater degrees of focal attention and concentration. It has also been established that positive treatment outcome is not always related to deep trance. In fact moderate depth of trance and other therapeutic variables (such as motivation and rapport) appear to be the most important factors determining positive treatment outcome (Hammond, 1998).

Nevertheless, certain behavioral, cognitive, perceptual and somatosensory changes are more likely to occur in deeper levels of hypnotic trance. Furthermore, greater perceived depth of trance can increase the responsiveness to treatment by ratifying trance experience, building positive expectancy, and increasing belief in the potency of the hypnotic intervention (Kirsch, 1990).

It is important to recognize that the depth of trance is not constant. Depth of trance can fluctuate both within and between sessions. Several factors such as the type of suggestions, external distractions, motivation, and amount of time used can affect the depth of trance (Hammond, 1998). It is therefore critical for the therapist to monitor the level of trance and deepen the trance as the need arises by offering suggestions for deepening the trance.

There are as many hypnotic deepening techniques as there are therapists. Hammond (1998) has listed 22 deepening techniques, including:

○ utilizing breathing and imagining internal relaxation

○ yogic breathing

○ contingent suggestions and utilizing patient behaviors

○ using ideomotor phenomena

○ progressive relaxation

○ fractionation

○ rapid fractionation

○ utilizing patient motivation and needs

○ downward movement

○ post-hypnotic suggestions and conditioning

○ visual imagery

○ periods of silence

○ breathing and counting

○ counting

○ metaphor for deepening despite background distractions

○ dual tasks

○ gently pushing the patient deeper

○ deepening by a series of graduated tasks

○ hand rotation or automatic movements

○ the metronome

○ confusional techniques

○ the revolving wheels fantasy.

Two deepening techniques – the counting technique and the downward movement technique – are described here.

The counting technique

There are different variations of the counting technique for deepening trance. In one variation the patient is asked to silently count a number each time they breathe in and out. The task can be made more complicated by asking the patient to rhythmically count backwards by twos or threes from 1000. The complicated counting overloads 'conscious spectatoring' and is particularly helpful when the patient is distracted by other stimuli such as noise or the presence of others, or when the patient believes he or she is not able to concentrate or focus on a task.

Another variation of the counting technique is for the therapist to count from one to five or one to ten and suggest that, with each count, the patient will experience deeper relaxation and deeper trance state:

> . . . now I am going to help you to feel even more relaxed. In order to do this I am going to count ONE to FIVE . . . When I reach the count of FIVE . . . at the count of FIVE . . . you will be resting in a deep . . . deep . . . very deep trance. (*See* Appendix 2A.)

Downward movement technique

With this deepening procedure, the patient is asked to imagine walking down a long staircase and, with each step, the patient experiences going into a deeper trance state. The image of an escalator or an elevator may also be used, but it will be important to ensure that the patient is not afraid of elevators or escalators. I usually use the image of a descending elevator for deepening the hypnotic trance.

THE DOWNWARD MOVEMENT TECHNIQUE

Imagine yourself being on the 10th floor of a large hotel. You are waiting for the elevator to arrive as you wish to go into the lobby on the first or main floor.

In a moment, as you imagine yourself descending down the elevator, you will become more and more relaxed, so that when you reach the main floor, you will be resting in deep, deep hypnotic trance.

Imagine the elevator has arrived, the doors open and two people get out. You get in the elevator and the doors close. You begin to feel the elevator is going down and you feel you are becoming more and more relaxed, more and more comfortable.

Now the elevator stops on the ninth floor, one person gets out and two persons get in. The doors close and the elevator begins to descend and you feel you are becoming more and more relaxed, more and more comfortable, drifting into a deep hypnotic state, so that when you reach the main floor you will be resting in a deep hypnotic trance. (*The idea behind noticing the number of people getting in and out of the elevator is to help the patient sustain focus and concentration.*)

The elevator does not stop on the eighth floor. It continues to descend and you are becoming more and more relaxed.

It stops on the seventh floor. The doors open and three people get out and two people come in. The doors close and the elevator begins to descend. You feel you are becoming more and more relaxed, drifting into a deep, deep hypnotic state.

It stops on the fifth floor. The doors open, no one gets out, two people come in. The doors close and the elevator begins to descend and you feel you are drifting into a deeper and deeper hypnotic state, so that when you reach the main floor you will be resting in a very deep, deep hypnotic trance.

The elevator stops on the fourth floor. The doors open and one person gets out and one person comes in. The doors close and it begins to move and you feel you are drifting into a very deep, deep trance.

It stops on the third floor. Three people get out and two people come in. The doors close and it begins to descend. Just notice how very relaxed you feel, becoming more and more comfortable drifting into a deep, deep trance.

The elevator does not stop on the second floor; it continues to descend and you feel you are drifting into a very deep, deep hypnotic trance. Feeling very, very relaxed, drifting into a deep, deep trance.

The elevator stops on the main floor and you feel you are in a very, very deep trance, drifting into a deep, deep hypnotic state.

The elevator technique can be extended to further deepen the trance. The patient can be given the suggestion to imagine walking down the corridor from the lobby into a quiet, cosy room, where the patient feels safe and secure, and can just let himself or herself drift into a very deep trance. Going down, the elevator technique can also be utilized to prepare the patient for age regression, where each floor represents an age.

STAGE 4: THERAPEUTIC UTILIZATION OF HYPNOSIS

As I have been stressing, hypnosis is not therapy. The induction and deepening of hypnosis do not produce lasting clinical benefits. Hypnosis is usually used as an adjunctive tool in the treatment of a variety of common psychiatric and medical problems. Maldonado and Spiegel (2003, p. 1294) argue that 'Because the hypnotic state involves an enhanced and altered state of concentration with an ability to produce changes in perception and certain body functions, it makes sense that it would be an effective tool in managing' such problems as depression, habit disorders, anxiety and phobic conditions, psychosomatic disorders and pain. A variety of hypnotic techniques, including ego-strengthening (*see* below), are used to help patients deal with their symptoms. Ego-strengthening provides positive reinforcement for behavior change (Crasilneck and Hall, 1985).

Hypnosis is also used as an adjunct to many types of psychotherapy, such as psychodynamic psychotherapy, behavior therapy, cognitive behavior therapy, gestalt therapy, group therapy, and marital therapy. However, the demarcation between psychotherapy and hypnotherapy is hard to identify because many psychotherapeutic techniques are ingrained within the hypnotic context. Some of these techniques include suggestive therapies, imagery training, visualization techniques, flooding, reframing, and double bind procedures. While these approaches are conceptually distinguishable from formal hypnosis, they are conventionally regarded as *hypnotic techniques* (Braun and Horevitz, 1986) and *hypnotherapy* refers to the utilization of hypnotic techniques throughout the course of treatment (Braun and Horevitz, 1986).

Hypnotic techniques can also facilitate abreaction and provide a vehicle for unconscious exploration and restructuring. In other words, hypnosis provides the context within which hypnotic strategies can be integrated with other therapeutic modalities to enhance treatment effect. There is some empirical evidence that when hypnosis is combined with other forms of psychotherapy in the treatment of emotional disorders, the outcome is enhanced. Kirsch *et al.* (1995) carried out a meta-analysis of 18 studies (1974 to 1993) comparing cognitive behavior therapy (CBT) with the same treatment supplemented by hypnosis to examine the additive effect of hypnosis in the management of various psychological disorders. Their review found the mean effect size was significantly larger for the treatment combined with hypnosis than for the non-hypnotic treatment.

More recently, Bryant *et al.* (2005) compared hypnosis plus CBT, CBT and supportive counselling with a group of patients with acute stress disorder. Hypnosis plus CBT was more effective than the other two options for re-experiencing symptoms at the end of treatment, but CBT and CBT + hypnosis were equivalent at six months and three-year follow-ups, and they were both better than supportive counselling at all three testing times with regard to post-traumatic stress disorder and depression symptomatology.

Bryant *et al.* (2005) speculated that the initial benefits of adding hypnosis to CBT might be retained if hypnosis were employed in additional ways rather than just imaginal exposure. Similarly, Alladin and Alibhai (2007) compared the effect of cognitive hypnotherapy (hypnosis combined with CBT) and CBT with 84 chronic depressives. At the end of the 16-week treatment, patients from both groups significantly improved compared to baseline scores. However, the cognitive hypnotherapy group produced significantly larger changes in Beck Depression Inventory (BDI-II), Beck Anxiety Inventory (BAI) and Beck Hopelessness Scale (BHS) scores. The effect size calculations showed that the cognitive hypnotherapy group produced 6%, 5% and 8% greater reduction in depression, anxiety and hopelessness, respectively, over and above the CBT group at the termination of treatment. The effect size was maintained at six-month and twelve-month follow-ups, demonstrating that the cognitive hypnotherapy group continued to improve after the termination of treatment.

There is accumulating evidence that high hypnotizability is associated with several serious psychiatric disorders (*see* Maldonado and Siegel, 2003 for a review). For example, the recent literature on dissociative identity disorder (previously known as multiple personality disorder) indicates that the majority of the patients with this disorder are highly hypnotizable and have a childhood history of severe physical and sexual abuse. This observation has led clinicians to recognize that the capacity to dissociate is mobilized both during and after extreme trauma. Hypnosis can be utilized to gain rapid access to these dissociative states and the process can be used to demonstrate to these patients how dissociation can be controlled.

Several studies have also found evidence (although other studies failed to replicate the finding) that phobic patients are highly hypnotizable compared to control populations (*see* Maldonado and Spiegel, 2003). From these findings, Maldonado and Spiegel (2003, pp. 1291–2) observe that 'it is possible that some kinds of phobic symptoms mobilize dissociative capacity, with the symptom representing absorption in the fear of the situation and suspension of critical judgment about it'. In recognition of these findings and observations, hypnosis can be utilized as an adjunct to the psychotherapy of phobic conditions to control the level of dissociation and suspension of critical judgement experienced by phobic patients.

Yapko (1992) has offered six clinical reasons for utilizing hypnosis with depression; hypnosis:

❍ amplifies subjective experience

❍ serves as a powerful method for interrupting symptomatic pattern

❍ facilitates experiential learning

❍ helps to bridge and conceptualize responses

❍ provides different models of inner reality

❍ helps to establish the focus of attention.

Chapters 4 and 5 describe in detail how hypnosis can be utilized effectively to treat migraine headache and depression. Chapter 3 briefly reviews the application of hypnosis in medicine and psychiatry.

Like any other treatment, not all patients or symptoms are amenable to hypnotherapy. Moreover, hypnotherapy may not be appropriate during all phases of treatment. However, there are no absolute guidelines or contraindications for utilizing hypnotherapy. Experience and clinical judgement serve as the deciding factors with each individual patient.

STAGE 5: EGO-STRENGTHENING

Most therapists focus on ego-strengthening prior to removing or modifying symptoms. The concept of 'ego-strengthening' was coined and popularized by Hartland (1971). The principle behind ego-strengthening, according to Hartland, is to remove tension, anxiety and apprehension, and to gradually restore the patient's confidence in him- or herself to cope with his or her problems. Hence his ego-strengthening suggestions consist of generalized supportive suggestions to increase the patient's confidence, coping abilities, positive self-image and interpersonal skills (*see* Appendix 2C). He points out that patients need to feel confident and strong enough to let go of the symptoms. Hartland recommends using ego-strengthening as a routine procedure in psychotherapy before direct removal of symptoms or hypnoanalysis, as this is likely to:

> . . . pay handsome dividends. Not only will the patient obtain more rapid relief from his symptoms, but he will display obvious improvements in other ways. You will notice him becoming more self-reliant, more confident and more able to adjust to his environment, and thus less prone to relapse. (Hartland, 1971, p. 197)

Bandura (1977) has provided experimental evidence that *self-efficacy* (the expectation and confidence to be able to cope successfully with various situations) is one of the key elements in the effective treatment of phobic disorders. Individuals with a sense of high self-efficacy tend to perceive themselves as being in control. If patients can be helped to view themselves as self-efficacious, they will perceive the future as being hopeful.

Torem (1990) regards ego-strengthening as analogous to the situation in the medical setting where a patient is first strengthened by proper nutrition, general rest and weight gain before being subjected to radical surgery. Alladin and Heap (1991, p. 58) consider ego-strengthening to be 'a way of exploiting the positive experience of hypnosis and the therapist–patient relationship in order to develop feelings of confidence and optimism and an improved self-image'. It is also believed that when ego-strengthening or positive suggestions are repeated to oneself, they become embedded in the unconscious mind and begin to exert automatic influence on feelings, thoughts and behavior (e.g. Hartland, 1971; Hammond, 1990; Heap and Aravind, 2002).

STAGE 6: POST-HYPNOTIC SUGGESTIONS

It is common practice to offer post-hypnotic suggestions before the termination of the hypnotic session. Post-hypnotic suggestions are given to counter problem behaviors, negative emotions, dysfunctional cognitions, and negative self-affirmations. Yapko (2003) regards post-hypnotic suggestions as a necessary part of the therapeutic process if the patient is to carry new possibilities into future experience, and many clinicians use post-hypnotic suggestions to shape behavior.

For example, Clarke and Jackson (1983) regard post-hypnotic suggestion as a form of 'higher-order-conditioning', which functions as positive or negative reinforcement to increase or decrease the probability of desired or undesired behaviors, respectively. They have successfully utilized post-hypnotic suggestions to enhance the effect of *in vivo* exposure among agoraphobics. Here is an example of the type of post-hypnotic suggestions that can be used to counter negative thinking in depression.

AN EXAMPLE OF POST-HYPNOTIC SUGGESTION

As a result of this treatment, as a result of you listening to your tape every day . . . every day you will become less preoccupied with yourself . . . less preoccupied with your feelings . . . and less preoccupied with what you think other people think about you. As a result of this, every day you will become more and more interested in what you are doing and what is going on around you.

STAGE 7: SELF-HYPNOSIS TRAINING

Modern hypnotherapy emphasizes the educational aspect of the hypnotic experience. In particular, 'It is most efficient to structure the intervention as a lesson in self-hypnosis that the patient can learn to employ in the service of symptom reduction' (Maldonado and Spiegel, 2003). At the end of the first hypnotherapy session, the patient is provided with an audiotape of self-hypnosis (consisting of the full script from Appendix 2C) designed to (a) create a good frame of mind, (b) offer ego-strengthening suggestions, and (c) provide post-hypnotic suggestions. The patient is encouraged to listen to the self-hypnosis tape daily and advised to adapt part of the self-hypnosis script to real-life situations. The homework assignment provides continuity of treatment between sessions and offers the patient the opportunity to learn self-hypnosis.

The self-hypnosis component of the therapy is specifically designed to create positive affect and counter negative self-talk. The ultimate goal of any form of psychotherapy is to help the patient establish self-reliance and independence. Alman (2001) believes patients can achieve self-reliance and personal power by learning self-hypnosis. Yapko (2003) contends that the teaching of self-hypnosis and problem-solving strategies to patients allows them to develop self-correcting mechanisms that give them control over their lives.

STAGE 8: TERMINATION OF HYPNOSIS

One of the most popular ways of terminating hypnosis is to count either one to five or five to one. The choice of numbers and whether to count up or down is purely arbitrary. What is important is that the patient is instructed. I normally count one to seven, and before counting I always state, 'In a moment . . . when I count from ONE to SEVEN you will open your eyes . . . and will be alert . . . without feeling tired . . . without feeling drowsy' (*see* Appendix 2A).

APPENDIX 2A

Cognitive hypnotherapy case formulation and treatment plan

Identifying Information:
Today's date:
Name:
Age:
Gender:
Marital status:
Ethnicity:
Occupational status:
Living situation:
Referred by:

1. Problem list:
(*List all major symptoms and problems in functioning.*)
Psychological/psychiatric symptoms:
Interpersonal difficulties:
Occupational problems:
Medical problems:
Financial difficulties:
Housing problems:
Legal issues:
Leisure problems:

2. Diagnosis:
Axis I:
Axis II:
Axis III:
Axis IV:
Axis V:

3. Working hypothesis:
(*Hypothesize the underlying mechanism producing the listed problems.*)
Assess schemas related to:
self:
other:

world:
future:
recurrent core beliefs:
rumination/negative self-hypnosis:
hypnotic suggestibility:

4. Precipitant/activating situations:
(*List triggers for current problems and establish connection between underlying mechanism and triggers of current problems.*)
Triggers:
Are triggers congruent with self-schemas/rumination/self-hypnosis?

5. Origins of core beliefs:
(*Establish origin of core beliefs from childhood experience.*)
Early adverse negative life events:
Genetic predisposition:
History of treatment (include response):

6. Summary of working hypothesis:
1.
2.
3.

7. Treatment plan:
1.
2.
3.
4.
Modality:
Frequency:
Interventions:
Adjunct therapies:
Obstacles:

8. Strengths and assets:
(*Based on the formulation, predict obstacles to treatment that may arise.*)
1.
2.
3.

APPENDIX 2B

Cognitive hypnotherapy case formulation and treatment plan for Cathy: a completed example for a patient with chronic depression

Identifying Information:
Today's Date: *February 10, 2006*
Name: *Cathy*
Age: *32 years old*
Gender: *Female*
Marital status: *Single*
Ethnicity: *White Caucasian*
Occupational status: *Paralegal assistant*
Living situation: *Lives on her own in a semi-detached house*
Referred by: *Dr. Spock, Psychiatrist*

1. Problem list:

(*List all major symptoms and problems in functioning.*)
Psychological/psychiatric symptoms:

Depressed, lacking energy, disturbed sleep, tired, and difficulty concentrating. She also experiences anxiety and inner tension, and finds it very difficult to unwind or relax. Occasional suicidal ideation, but no intent or plan for suicide.

Interpersonal difficulties:

Withdrawn, avoids friends, social contacts and social functions. She has good interpersonal skills and she has several close women friends, but keeps away from them. She has been divorced for 5 years and since then she has not dated. She lacks confidence dating and she believes she cannot trust me.

Occupational problems:

She works as a paralegal assistant in a very busy law office, consisting of 18 people, including lawyers, paralegal assistants and secretarial staff. She likes her job. Her ambition was to become a lawyer, but since her divorce she feels she has no confidence to go to university.

Medical problems:
    None

Financial difficulties:
    None

Housing problems:
    None

Legal issues:
    None

Leisure problems:
    She avoids social interaction because she feels she lacks confidence and derives no pleasure being with other people. She believes she is no longer the extrovert she used to be. She believes her ex-husband has taken away her confidence and made her become a 'no one'.

2. Diagnosis:

Axis I: *Major depressive disorder, recurrent, moderate*
Axis II: *None*
Axis III: *None*
Axis IV: *Divorced; socially isolated; lonely.*
Axis V: *GAF score = 50*

3. Working hypothesis:

(Hypothesize the underlying mechanism producing the listed problems.)
Assess schemas related to:
Self:
    'I am no one.'
    'I have no confidence.'
    'He destroyed me; he took away my pride and my dignity.'
    'He turned me into a failure; he took away my personality.'

Other:
    'You can't trust anyone; people are so mean, they exploit you.'
    'It's not worth having a relationship; it only brings pain.'

World:

'The world is selfish and uncaring.'

'There are too many problems and obstacles, you can never succeed so what's the point in trying.'

Future:

'I don't have a future; he destroyed everything.'

'I see myself unhappy and struggling for the rest of my life.'

'I see myself being lonely and isolated for the rest of my life.'

Recurrent core beliefs:

'I am useless; he took away everything and turned me into a failure.'

'I can never be the same person again.'

Rumination/negative self-hypnosis:

She ruminates on the beliefs that her husband (who was alcoholic and emotionally and physically abusive to her) has destroyed her personality and turned her into a failure. She believes she has no confidence and therefore she will not be able to achieve anything in her life.

Hypnotic suggestibility:

She scored maximum on the Babrer Suggestibility Scale.

4. Precipitant/activating situations:

(*List triggers for current problems and establish connection between underlying mechanism and triggers of current problems.*)

Triggers:

Being alone in her house; attending social functions; holidays and festive seasons.

Are triggers congruent with self-schemas/rumination/self-hypnosis?

The triggers activate her self-schema of being a failure and lacking confidence. Therefore she will not be able to do anything.

5. Origins of core beliefs:

(*Establish origin of core beliefs from childhood's experience.*)

Early adverse negative life-events:

She was brought up in a stressful home environment. Her father was an alcoholic and physically aggressive to her mother. As a child, on several occasions, she witnessed her father hitting her mother. She was scared of her father. She had very little love and attention from her father. However, her mother was very caring and attentive to her needs and protected her against her father. Cathy felt helpless that she was not able to help and protect her mother. She was therefore dependent on her mother for her sense of security and emotional needs.

Genetic predisposition:

Cathy's grandmother had a history of major depressive disorder. Since childhood Cathy had the tendency to think very negatively about herself.

History of treatment (include response):

Followed-up by a psychiatrist for 5 years. Tried several antidepressant medications, but none had worked for her.

6. Summary of working hypothesis:

Whenever Cathy is at home on her own, she feels lonely. This feeling triggers the thoughts that her husband has destroyed her personality and her self-esteem. These negative cognitions are also triggered whenever she is invited to attend a social function or whenever a festive season is imminent. These negative cognitions revive her self-schemas that she is a failure, resulting in feeling anxious and depressed. Rumination of these feelings intensify her affect and from this she concludes that she will never succeed in life.

7. Strengths and assets:

Stable job and lifestyle; bright; excellent social skills; has friends.

8. Treatment plan:

Goals (measures):

1. Reduce anxiety and depressive symptoms, which can be monitored via the BDI-II and the BAI.
2. Reduce procrastination, which can be monitored via log of activities.
3. Increase social activities and social contacts (measured via number of contacts).
4. Begin dating in an effort to meet husband (measured via number of dates).
5. Find information about admission to law schools and meet counselor from the local university to discuss admission and career planning.

6. Sign up with the local gym and work out at least three times a week.

Modality:
  Individual cognitive hypnotherapy.

Frequency:
  Weekly for 10 weeks.

Interventions:
  Teach the formulation (to provide rationale for interventions).
  Activity scheduling (gym, socializing, dating, exploring admission to law school).
  Cognitive restructuring (RET-Worksheet, behavioral experiments).
  Ego-strengthening for increasing self-esteem.
  Schema change interventions.

Adjunct therapies:
  Medication will be considered as an option if she does not respond to cognitive hypnotherapy.

Obstacles:
  Procrastination, low self-esteem, and too focused on the past hurts.

APPENDIX 2C
Hypnotic induction relaxation with counting method

This script also contains deepening, termination and ego-strengthening suggestions.

Close your eyes and make yourself as comfortable as you can. Now I am going to count ONE to TEN . . . As I count . . . with every count you will become more and more relaxed . . . so that when I reach the count of 10 . . . at the count of 10 you will be resting in a deep trance.

ONE: Just continue to breathe gently . . . in and out . . . and as you concentrate on my voice you begin to relax . . . relaxing very deeply as you continue to listen to my voice.

TWO: You begin to feel a heavy and relaxing feeling coming over you as you continue to listen to my voice . . . And as you continue to breathe in and out . . . you will begin to feel your arms relaxing . . . your legs relaxing . . . your entire body relaxing completely.

THREE: You begin to feel that heavy and relaxing feeling beginning to increase . . . more and more . . . and you are beginning to relax . . . more and more . . . relaxing deeper and deeper all the time as you continue to listen to my voice.

FOUR: You can feel that heavy and relaxing feeling increasing . . . more and more as you continue to listen to my voice . . . .. And as I continue to count, with every count . . . that heavy and relaxing feeling will continue to increase more and more . . . until they cause you to drift into a deep and pleasant trance.

FIVE: Just notice . . . progressively you are becoming more and more relaxed . . . more and more at ease . . . more and more comfortable . . . so that when I reach the count of TEN, you will be resting in a deep trance.

SIX: Just listen to my voice as I continue to count . . . and by the time I get to the count of TEN . . . you will be resting in a deep and pleasant trance.

SEVEN: You are beginning to drift slowly into a deep . . . deep trance.

EIGHT: Just notice you are becoming more and more comfortable . . . more and more at ease . . . more and more deeply relaxed . . . so that when I reach the count of TEN, you will be resting in a deep trance.

NINE: And every time you breathe in and out . . . you are drifting slowly into a deep and pleasant trance . . . drifting slowly . . . into a deep and pleasant trance.

TEN: Drifting slowly into a deep trance as you continue to listen to my voice . . . as you continue to breathe in and out . . . drifting deeper . . . and deeper . . . down . . . and down . . . into a deep and pleasant trance.

Creating a pleasant state of mind

After the initial induction, it is advisable to spend a few minutes to enhance the relaxation and the 'good' feeling before deepening the trance. The enhancement of the good feeling creates a pleasant state of mind, which helps to ratify the trance, thus preparing the patient for the deepening suggestions.

CREATING A PLEASANT STATE OF MIND

You have now become so deeply relaxed . . . and you are in such a deep . . . deep trance . . . that your mind and your body feel completely relaxed . . . completely at ease. You begin to feel a beautiful sensation of peace and relaxation . . . tranquility and calm . . . flowing through your mind and body. You feel this beautiful sensation of peace and relaxation, tranquility and calm . . . flowing all over your mind and body . . . giving you such a pleasant feeling . . . such a soothing feeling . . . that you feel completely relaxed . . . completely at ease. Your mind and your body feel completely relaxed . . . and perfectly at ease . . . feeling calm . . . peaceful . . . comfortable . . . completely relaxed . . . totally relaxed . . . drifting into a deeper and deeper trance as you continue to listen to my voice.

Deepening the trance

Once the patient is prepared for deep trance through the creation of the pleasant state of mind, the simplest deepening technique can deepen the trance. I normally use the counting method of deepening the trance.

DEEPENING THE TRANCE

You are in such a deep hypnotic trance now . . . that your mind and your body feel calm and peaceful. And now I am going to help you to feel even more relaxed. In order to do this I am going to count ONE to FIVE . . . When I reach the count of FIVE . . . at the count of FIVE . . . you will be resting in a deep . . . deep . . . very deep trance.

ONE . . . just let yourself go . . . just let yourself relax . . .

TWO . . . not doing anything . . . not trying anything . . . just letting go . . . no efforts . . . effortless.

THREE . . . becoming heavier and heavier . . . [or lighter and lighter] . . . sinking deeper and deeper into a deep, deep trance. (*From the administration of a standardized suggestibility test and/or from the initial hypnotic induction, the therapist will be aware of the kind of sensations, e.g. light, heavy or detached, that the patient is prone to feel. These sensations can be reinforced while inducing a deep trance.*)

FOUR . . . feeling heavier and heavier . . . [or lighter and lighter] . . . and at the same time feeling detached. Feeling very, very detached . . . your whole body feeling completely detached . . . drifting into a deeper and deeper trance.

FIVE . . . letting yourself drift into a deeper and deeper trance . . . drifting deeper and deeper as you continue to listen to my voice.

EGO-STRENGTHENING SUGGESTIONS

Just continue to enjoy these beautiful feelings . . . and as you continue to enjoy this feeling of deep relaxation . . . I am going to repeat some helpful and positive suggestions to you . . . and since you are very relaxed and in such a deep hypnotic trance . . . your mind has become so sensitive . . . so receptive to what I say . . . so that every suggestion that I give you . . . will sink so deeply into the unconscious part of your mind . . . that they will begin to cause such a lasting impression there . . . that nothing will eradicate them . . . These suggestions from within your unconscious mind will help you resolve your difficulties . . . They will help you with your thinking . . . that is, they will help you to think more clearly, more objectively, more realistically, and more positively . . . They will help you with your feelings . . . that is, they will make you feel less anxious, less upset, less depressed . . . They will also help you with your actions and your behaviors . . . that is, they will help you to do more and more things that are helpful to you, and you will do fewer and fewer things that are not helpful to you.

You are now so deeply relaxed, you are in such deep hypnotic trance . . . that everything that I say will happen to you . . . for your own good . . . will happen more and more . . . And every feeling that I tell you that you will experience . . . you will begin to experience more and more . . . These same things will happen to you more and more often as you listen to your tape . . . And the same things will begin to happen to you just as strongly . . . just as powerfully . . . when you are at home . . . or at work or at school . . . or in any situation that you may find yourself in.

You are now so deeply relaxed . . . you are in such a deep hypnotic trance . . . that you are going to feel physically stronger and fitter in every way. At the end of the session . . . and every time you listen to your tape . . .you will feel more alert . . . more wide awake . . . more energetic . . . Every day as you learn to relax . . . you will become much less easily tired . . . much less easily fatigued . . . much less easily discouraged . . . much less easily upset . . . much less easily depressed.

Therefore every day as you learn to relax . . . your mind and your body will feel physically stronger and healthier . . . your nerves will become stronger and steadier . . . your mind will become calmer and clearer . . . you will feel more composed . . . more relaxed . . . and able to let go . . . You will begin to develop the tendency to ruminate less . . . to catastrophize less . . . therefore, you will become less worried . . . less anxious and less apprehensive . . . less easily upset . . . less easily depressed.

As you become more relaxed, less anxious and less worried every day . . . you will begin to take more and more interest in whatever you are doing . . . in whatever is going on around you . . . that your mind will become completely distracted away from yourself . . . You will no longer think nearly so much about yourself . . . you will no longer dwell nearly so much on yourself and your difficulties . . . and you will become much less conscious of yourself . . . much less preoccupied with yourself and your difficulties . . . much less preoccupied with your own feelings . . . and much less preoccupied with what you think others think of you.

As you become less preoccupied with yourself, less conscious of yourself . . . you will be able to think more clearly . . . you will be able to concentrate more easily . . . You will be able to give your whole undivided attention to whatever you are doing . . . to the complete exclusion of everything else . . . Even if some thoughts cross your mind, you will be able to concentrate on the task without being distracted . . . As a result of this, your memory will begin to improve . . . so that you begin to see things in their true perspective . . . without magnifying your difficulties . . . without ever allowing them to get out of proportion . . . In other words, from now on . . . whenever you have a problem, you will examine it objectively and realistically . . . and decide what you can and cannot do about it . . . If you cannot resolve the problem . . . you will accept it and come to terms with it . . . But if the problem can be resolved . . . then you will make a plan . . . or come up with some strategies to overcome it however long it may take . . . Therefore from now on . . . whenever you have a problem you will become less emotionally upset and less overwhelmed by it . . . From now on you will begin to examine your difficulties like a scientist, that is, taking everything into consideration and then coming up with a plan . . . As a result of this new attitude . . . you will become emotionally less upset . . . less anxious . . . less agitated . . . and less depressed.

Every day . . . you will begin to feel all these things happening . . . more and more rapidly . . . more and more powerfully . . . more and more completely . . . so that . . . you will feel much happier . . . much more contented . . . much more optimistic in every way. And you will gradually become much more able to rely upon . . . to depend upon yourself . . . your own efforts . . . your own judgement . . . your own opinions . . . In fact . . . you will begin to feel much less need . . . to rely upon . . . or to depend . . . upon . . . other people.

Post-hypnotic suggestions

TERMINATION

Now . . . for the next few moments just let yourself relax completely . . . and continue to feel this beautiful sensation of peace . . . and relaxation . . . tranquility . . . and calm . . . flowing through your entire body . . . giving you such a pleasant . . . such a soothing sensation . . . that you feel so good . . . so at ease . . . that you feel a sense of well-being.

In a moment . . . when I count from ONE to SEVEN you will open your eyes . . . and will be alert . . . without feeling tired . . . without feeling drowsy . . . You will feel much better for this deep and pleasant hypnotic experience . . . You will feel completely relaxed both mentally and physically . . . and you will feel confident both in yourself and the future.

Now I am going to count ONE to SEVEN . . . ONE . . . TWO . . . THREE . . . FOUR . . . FIVE . . . SIX . . . SEVEN . . . Open your eyes . . . feeling relaxed, refreshed, and a sense of well-being.

REFERENCES

Alladin A. (2007). *Handbook of Cognitive Hypnotherapy for Depression: an evidence-based approach*. Philadelphia: Lippincott Williams and Wilkins.

Alman, B. (2001). Self-care: approaches from self-hypnosis for utilizing your unconscious (inner) potentials. In Greary B, Zeig J, editors. *The Handbook of Ericksonian Psychotherapy* (pp. 522–40). Phoenix, AZ: Milton H. Erickson Foundation Press.

American Psychiatric Association. (2000). *Diagnostic and Statistical Manual of Mental Disorders*. 4th ed. Washington, DC: American Psychiatric Association.

Araoz DL. (1981). Negative self-hypnosis. *Journal of Contemporary Psychotherapy* 12: 45–52.

Araoz DL. (1985). *The New Hypnosis*. New York: Brunner/Mazel.

Bandura, A. (1977). *Self-efficacy: the exercise of control*. New York: Freeman.

Barabasz A, Watkins JG. (2005). *Hypnotherapeutic Techniques*. 2nd ed. New York: Brunner-Routledge.

Beck AT, Steer RA. (1993a). *Beck Anxiety Inventory*. San Antonio, TX: Harcourt Brace.

Beck AT, Steer RA. (1993b). *Beck Hopelessness Scale*. San Antonio, TX: Harcourt Brace.

Beck AT, Steer RA, Brown KB. (1996). *The Beck Depression Inventory — Revised*. San Antonio, TX: Harcourt Brace.

Beutler LE, Clarkin JE, Bongar B. (2000). *Guidelines for the Systematic Treatment of the Depressed Patient*. New York: Oxford University Press.

Clarke JC, Jackson JA. (1983). *Hypnosis and Behavior Therapy: the treatment of anxiety and phobias*. New York: Springer.

Golden WL, Dowd ET, Friedberg F. (1987). *Hypnotherapy: a modern approach*. New York: Pergamon Press.

Hammond DC, editor. (1990). *Hypnotic Induction and Suggestions*. Chicago, Illinois: American Society of Clinical Hypnosis.

Hartland J. (1971). *Medical and Dental Hypnosis and its Clinical Applications*. 2nd ed. London: Bailliere Tindall.

Ledley DR, Marx BP, Heimberg RG. (2005). *Making Cognitive-Behavioral Therapy Work: clinical process for new practitioners*. New York: Guilford Press.

Lynn SJ, Kirsch I. (2006). *Essentials of Clinical Hypnosis: an evidence-based approach*. Washington, DC: American Psychological Association.

Needleman LD. (2003). Case conceptualization in preventing and responding to therapeutic difficulties. In: Leahy RL, editor. *Roadblocks in Cognitive-behavioral Therapy: transforming challenges into opportunities for change* (pp. 3–23). New York: Guilford Press.

Persons JB, Davidson J, Tompkins MA. (2001). *Essential Components of Cognitive-behavior Therapy for Depression*. Washington, DC: American Psychological Association.

Torem, MS. (1990). Ego strengthening. In: Hammond DC, editor. Handbook of Hypnotic Suggestions and Metaphors. (pp. 110–2). New York: Norton.

Warren WL. (1994). *Revised Hamilton Rating Scale for Depression (RHRSD): manual.* Los Angeles: Western Psychological Services.

World Health Organization. (1992). *Tenth Revision of the International Classification of Diseases.* Geneva: World Health Organization.

Yapko M. (1995). *Essentials of Hypnosis.* New York: Brunner/Mazel Publishers.

Yapko MD. (2003). *Trancework: an introduction to the practice of clinical hypnosis.* 3rd ed. New York: Brunner-Routledge.

CHAPTER 3

Hypnotherapy as an Intervention in Medicine and Psychiatry

SUMMARY

This chapter reviews the application of hypnosis to five medical conditions and five psychiatric disorders. The review demonstrates the effectiveness of hypnosis as an adjunct treatment with a variety of conditions, although some of the hypnotic applications require further empirical validation. The application of hypnosis to cancer appears to be challenging and daunting.

INTRODUCTION

This chapter discusses the application of hypnosis to medicine and psychiatry. The review indicates the close relationship between medicine – especially the field of psychiatry – and hypnosis in the development of the art and science of healing. Some specific medical and psychiatric disorders are selectively reviewed to illustrate the role of hypnosis as an effective adjunct treatment.

Hypnosis provided an alternative model of psychopathology in the 19th century, particularly in the understanding of dissociative and somatoform disorders. Mesmer, who is known as the father of modern hypnosis (although he did not strictly utilize hypnosis), is also credited as being the originator of the new field of talking therapy: psychotherapy (Ellenberger, 1970).

THE APPLICATION OF HYPNOSIS IN MEDICINE

Hypnosis has been used, in one form or other, to relieve pain and suffering since prehistoric times. 'Modern hypnosis' (Conn, 1957) dates back to the work of Franz Anton Mesmer, an Austrian physician, in the 18th century. Mesmer theorized that all objects were subject to magnetic fields that directly influence health and disease. He 'magnetized' his patient by making physical passes over their body; that is, he transmitted his own magnetic field in an attempt to restore equilibrium to his patient's 'magnetic fluid'. During this process the patient would have a seizure.

In 1774 Mesmer's claims that he was able to cure patients by restoring their magnetic fluid were investigated by a scientific commission appointed by Louis XVI of France. The commission was headed by Benjamin Franklin and consisted of many distinguished figures, including Antoine Lavoisier and Joseph-Ignace Guillotin. The commission concluded that Mesmer was a fake and that there was no evidence of magnetic fluid. Nevertheless, Mesmer cured many of his patients, and the commission attributed the cure to imagination and suggestion, not to the effect of the attributed 'magnetic fluid'.

In the 1800s the interest in medical hypnosis was revived by John Elliotson, a British physician, who was a noted professor of medicine and editor of *The Lancet*. Unfortunately, Elliotson got involved in mesmerism and phrenology and was eventually discredited by his medical colleagues. Another noted physician who advocated the medical use of hypnosis was James Esdaile. Esdaile used hypnosis to induce anesthesia in his surgical patients. It is reported that he carried out 1000 minor and 300 major medical–surgical procedures (Wain, 1980).

Another prominent British surgeon, James Braid, became interested in hypnosis in the 1840s, and he coined the word 'hypnotism' to describe hypnosis as a sleep-like state. Later Braid became more aware of the role of suggestibility and imagination in hypnosis (Gibson and Heap, 1991). Other prominent physicians of the 1800s who became interested in hypnosis were Jean-Martin Charcot, Pierre Janet, Sigmund Freud, Josef Breuer and Hippolyte Bernheim. They all used hypnosis very successfully, except for Freud, who rejected hypnosis and went on to develop psychoanalysis. In 1955 hypnosis was accepted as a valid medical concept by the British Medical Association, and in 1958 by the American Medical Association.

A review of the well-controlled empirical studies on the role of hypnosis in the treatment of a variety of medical conditions has provided convincing evidence for the clinical efficacy of hypnosis (Lynn *et al.*, 2000; Pinnell and Covino, 2000). The effectiveness of hypnosis in the management of pain has been even more remarkable. Hypnosis has an impressive history in the treatment of pain, beginning with reports in the mid-1800s (Esdaile, 1846/1976; Elliotson, 1843) of major surgeries that were performed with hypnosis as the sole anesthesia. A meta-analysis of controlled trials of hypnotic analgesia has demonstrated that hypnotherapy can provide relief for 75% of the patients studied (Montgomery *et al.*, 2000). The treatment was most effective for the patients who were highly suggestible to hypnosis. Other comprehensive reviews of the clinical trial literature indicate that hypnotherapy is effective with both acute and chronic pain (Elkins *et al.*, 2007; Patterson and Jensen, 2003).

Hypnotic intervention with medical patients can be an effective tool in addressing the suffering component, and it can facilitate a sense of control and self-mastery that promotes physiological as well as psychological equilibrium. Untreated psychological comorbidity with medical illness results in poorer physical health, less effective medical treatment and management, increased utilization of services, and increased costs of medical services (e.g. Katon *et al.*, 2002).

Five medical conditions – pain, respiratory disorders, gastrointestinal disorders, dermatological disorders and cancer – are reviewed in this chapter to demonstrate the effectiveness of hypnotherapy. The effectiveness of hypnosis in acute medical settings is also explored. Chapter 4 provides a detailed description of the 'prototype' of hypnotherapy for migraine headache.

Pain

The National Institutes of Health Technology Assessment Panel on Integration of Behavioral and Relaxation Approaches into the Treatment of Chronic Pain and Insomnia reviewed outcome studies on hypnosis with pain and concluded that research strongly supports the evidence that hypnosis is effective with chronic pain (National Institutes of Health, 1996). Similarly, a meta-analysis review of contemporary research on hypnosis and pain management (Montgomery *et al.*, 2000) reported that hypnosis meets the American Psychological Association criteria (Chambless and Hollon, 1998) for being an efficacious and specific treatment for pain, showing superiority over medication, psychological placebos and other treatments.

More recently, Elkins *et al.*, (2007) reviewed 13 controlled prospective trials of hypnosis for the treatment of chronic pain, which compared outcomes from hypnosis for the treatment of chronic pain with either baseline data or a control condition. The data indicate that hypnosis interventions consistently produce significant decreases in pain associated with a variety of chronic pain problems, including cancer, low back problems, arthritis, sickle cell disease, temporomandibular conditions, fibromyalgia, physical disability, and mixed etiologies (e.g. 15 lumbar pain, 7 rheumatological pain, 3 cervical pain, 1 peripheral neuropathy, 1 gynecological-related pain (the numbers refer to number of patients within each condition)).

Hypnosis was also generally found to be more effective than non-hypnotic interventions, such as attention, physical therapy and education. Most of the hypnosis interventions for chronic pain include instructions in self-hypnosis. However, there is a lack of standardization among the hypnotic interventions examined in clinical trials, and the number of patients enrolled in the studies has tended to be low and lacking long-term follow-up.

Similarly, Hammond (2007), from his review of the literature on the effectiveness of hypnosis in the treatment of headaches and migraines, concluded that hypnotherapy meets the clinical psychology research criteria for being a well-established and efficacious treatment for tension and migraine headaches. Hammond pointed out that hypnotherapy 'is virtually free of the side effects, risks of adverse reactions, and ongoing expense associated with medication treatments' (p. 207). Chapter 4 describes in detail a standard hypnotherapy protocol for treating migraine headache.

Respiratory disorders

Hypnosis has been used with a variety of respiratory and pulmonary disorders.

Brown (2007, in press), from his critical review of the controlled outcome studies of hypnotherapy for asthma, concludes that:

> There is no question that hypnosis has been shown across numerous studies to have beneficial effects on the subjective aspects of asthma, which include: symptom frequency and severity; coping with asthma-specific fears; managing acute attacks; and frequency of medication use and health visits. These effects include both genuine changes in illness-related behaviors as well as significant changes in the subjective appraisal of symptoms. In that sense, hypnotic treatment of asthma is clinically efficacious.

Similarly, Covino and Frankel (1993) concur in their review of the use of hypnosis and relaxation for medical conditions that:

> . . . several controlled studies demonstrate that hypnosis is more effective than relaxation or medication alone in the relief of symptoms . . . [and] those asthmatics with higher levels of hypnotizability seem to be most helped by hypnosis (p. 79).

However, Brown (2007) stresses the need for replication of research with better designs, larger samples and more careful attention paid to the types of suggestions given or strategies used in hypnosis.

When working with asthmatic patients, the focus is on teaching patients to:

> . . . learn to use self-hypnotic techniques rather than medication when they begin to feel an anxiety-precipitated asthmatic attack coming on. This may help interrupt the vicious cycle of anxiety and bronchoconstriction. (Maldonado and Spiegel, 2003, p. 1310).

Another common technique is to instruct asthmatic patients in self-hypnosis, which involves imagining being in an environment where they can breathe naturally and effortlessly (Spiegel and Spiegel, 1987).

Gastrointestinal disorders

Gastrointestinal (GI) disorders include disorders of the upper GI tract (diffuse esophageal spasm, reflux esophagitis, achalasia and peptic ulcer) and disorders of the lower GI tract (irritable bowel syndrome and inflammatory bowel disease).

Irritable bowel syndrome (IBS), which affects between 50 and 70% of all patients with GI symptoms (Brown and Fromm, 1986), has been extensively studied in the context of hypnotherapy. In 2006 a whole issue of the *International Journal of Clinical and Experimental Hypnosis* (January 2006, 54(1): 1–112) was devoted to IBS. This special issue provides readers with a complete overview of the evidence for the effectiveness of hypnosis treatment of IBS. It also gives an in-depth look at the two well-defined and successful hypnosis treatment paradigms for IBS that have been repeatedly tested in empirical studies – the approach of the Manchester group in England and the North Carolina standardized protocol. The issue also includes a thorough examination of the efforts by researchers to understand the mechanisms that can account for the therapeutic impact of hypnosis on IBS, new information on a case series of IBS patients treated with hypnosis, and pilot research on a home treatment application of hypnosis for the disorder.

Whithead (2006) reviewed 11 studies, including five controlled studies, to assess the therapeutic effects of hypnosis for IBS. Although this literature displays significant limitations, such as small sample sizes and lack of parallel comparisons with other treatments, this body of research consistently shows hypnosis to have a very substantial therapeutic impact in IBS, even for patients who have been unresponsive to standard medical interventions. The median response rate to hypnosis treatment is 87%, and therapeutic gains (reduction in abdominal pain, constipation and flatulence) are well maintained for most patients for years after the end of treatment.

The 'gut-directed hypnotherapy' developed by the Department of Medicine at the University Hospital of South Manchester, UK, is outlined below to provide a flavor of the adjunctive hypnotic techniques used with IBS. The gut-directed hypnotherapy consists of 12 weekly sessions of individual therapy with the same therapist over a three-month period. The basic components are:

○ patients becoming familiar with hypnosis and the treatment setting

○ when in trance, patients are reminded that they are learning relaxation skills, tapping their minds (conscious and unconscious) to learn to regulate the gut, and promoting balance in their bodily functions

○ practicing self-hypnosis via audiocassette or CD to promote inner calmness and relaxation

○ learning specific hypnotic techniques (e.g. warming the gut, imagining a normal gut, to control and normalize the gut function)

○ imaginal rehearsal of coping with situations that were avoided before

○ post-hypnotic suggestions of gaining control over the gut and reducing the symptoms.

Dermatological disorders

Hypnosis has been found to be helpful in a variety of dermatological conditions, in particular pruritus, eczema, acne, neurodermatitis, scleroderma, warts and psoriasis. Although dermatological disorders are mostly caused by bacteria, fungus, allergens, external stimuli and internal biochemical balance in the skin, and emotional stress (Barabasz and Watkins, 2005), recent scientific studies point to the role of stress in the onset and/or exacerbation of many dermatological problems (Hawkins, 2006).

Skin disorders are also associated with shame and embarrassment, and in turn can produce a host of psychological reactions such as anxiety, depression and social withdrawal. Hypnotherapeutic techniques, particularly ego-strengthening, can be utilized to deal with these psychological factors. In addition, some dermatologic conditions can be aggravated and maintained by secondary inflammation, infection, or lichenification caused by rubbing, scratching or picking. These secondary complications can be reduced by hypnotic interventions, thus promoting healing of the skin.

The script detailed below, which I use with acne, exemplifies the types of hypnotic suggestions that can be utilized when treating skin disorders with hypnosis. The script can be adapted for use with a variety of skin conditions. Following hypnotic induction, deepening and ego-strengthening, the image of taking a warm shower can be used. This procedure conveys the image of cleaning the unhealthy skin and promoting growth of new, healthy skin. The image of the warm shower also creates a sense of comfort, thus alleviating the irritation and the itching of the skin. Suggestions for emotional regulation are incorporated in the script to promote emotional regulation and balance.

USING HYPNOSIS TO TREAT ACNE

As you remain deeply relaxed, I want you to imagine having a warm shower. Imagine the warm water is flowing over your face, flowing over the affected areas of your face and other affected areas of your body. Feel the warm water gently moving and spreading over all the affected areas of your body.

Imagine you are gently massaging the affected areas while the warm water is flowing . . . and the warm water is producing a sense of comfort, easing away the irritation, easing away the tenderness, easing away the rash bumps, and allowing the skin to heal up. As the comfort spreads over all the affected areas, imagine the underlying texture of the skin is changing, is softening, and becoming more and more normal. You feel your skin is changing and becoming more relaxed, feeling more comfortable, feeling normal.

Continue to imagine gently rubbing the warm water to the affected areas until you feel a sense of complete comfort and relief. Your unconscious mind knows that this has influenced your skin sufficiently so that you will be able to maintain several hours of comfort. And within a minute or two you will become consciously aware of the comfort, and then you may awaken, realizing that you can apply this warm water again in self-hypnosis, whenever you need to.

As you imagine the warm water flowing and spreading over your skin, you feel the irritation, the discomfort, the tenderness and the rash bumps dissipating. As the tenderness and discomfort leave, the skin energy is left to continue the healing . . . Feel the active healing as the new cells on the surface of your skin replace the injured, irritated cells . . . Imagine the blood circulation below your skin is increasing and bringing in more oxygen and nutrition to nourish the healthy tissue growing on the skin.

Let this soothing and healing continue even after you open your eyes, for as long as possible . . . Each time you repeat this exercise, the post-exercise effect of warming and healing will continue a bit longer. Soon you will not need the exercise, as the healing will be complete.

Emotional upsets cause irritation of the nervous system, which in turn can affect the skin condition. This can lead to the redness and swelling of the skin condition. Continual irritation of the nervous system also affects the activity of the sweat glands, which may result in dysregulation of the sweat gland. The oiliness and dryness of the acne are caused by the dysregulation of the sweat gland, which may encourage the bacteria and the fungi in your skin to grow. All these factors can affect the blood flow to the skin, which contributes to the inflammation and irritation of the skin.

By listening to the self-hypnosis tape you will be able to produce a deep sense of relaxation. By relaxing your nervous system you are able to restore proper balance to its functioning and therefore the blood flow to your skin and the activity of the sweat glands are properly regulated.

As a result of this treatment . . . you are going to feel stronger and fitter in every way. Your circulation will improve . . . particularly the circulation through the little blood-vessels that supply the skin. Your heart will beat more strongly . . . so that more blood will flow through the little blood vessels in the skin . . . carrying more nourishment to the skin. Because of this . . . your skin will become much better nourished . . . it will become healthier . . . more normal in texture . . . and the rash will gradually diminish . . . until it fades away completely . . . leaving the underlying new skin perfectly healthy and normal in every respect.

Cancer

Apart from utilizing hypnotic techniques to deal with the secondary effects of cancer – pain, anxiety, depression, feelings of hopelessness, etc. – hypnosis has been used in the treatment of carcinomas (Barabasz and Watkins, 2005). The defining research in this area was conducted by David Spiegel and his colleagues (Kogan *et al.*, 1997) at Stanford University Medical School. In a randomized clinical trial, 50 of 85 women with metastatic breast cancer were offered weekly self-hypnosis and behavior therapy, and they were followed-up for 10 years. The patients who received this treatment had 50% less pain and survived a year and a half longer than did the patients who had standard medical care. Hypnotic visualization and imagery techniques have also been used to treat cancer directly and to control the side-effects of cancer therapy (Rosenberg, 1982–83). In treating cancer directly:

> The patient's motivation is stimulated by direct hypnotic suggestion. The aim of hypnosis is to mobilize the patient's own physical resources to fight the cancer.
>
> Imagery can involve visualizing the cancer in a form of the patient's own choosing. It might be perceived as a black mass, or perhaps symbolically as a castle that is being attacked. In a direct or symbolic manner, this cancer will be attacked by the patient's own powerful antibodies, and these patients will 'bite away' pieces of the cancer and imagine these pieces being carried away by their own normal eliminative processes. (Barabasz and Watkins, 2005, p. 305)

Although it is unlikely that psychological intervention will ever replace surgical, pharmacological and radiological treatments of cancer, it is important to explore different ways cancer patients can learn to strengthen their natural physiological resistances to neoplastic development. Given that hypnosis can alter physiological processes (*see* Chapter 1) and the immune system (Ruzyla-Smith *et al.*, 1995), further studies on the effect of hypnosis on cancer are warranted.

USE OF HYPNOSIS IN THE ACUTE MEDICAL SETTING

Hypnotic techniques have also been proven to be effective in the acute medical setting. For example, Lang *et al.* (1996), in a randomized trial, demonstrated that the use of hypnosis in interventional radiology produced better analgesia than that resulting from patient-controlled analgesia with midazolam and fentanyl, resulting in less anxiety, fewer side-effects, and fewer procedural interventions.

This finding was confirmed and replicated by Lang *et al.* (2000) with a larger prospective randomized trial involving 241 patients undergoing radiological interventions in the kidneys and vascular system. The patients were randomized to standard care, structured attention, or self-hypnotic relaxation and all received local anesthesia. Hypnosis significantly reduced pain, anxiety, drug use and complications. Moreover, the procedure time was 17 minutes shorter compared to the standard group. Time savings in combination with fewer complications resulted in a higher cost effectiveness compared to standardized treatments; savings were on average $330 per procedure (Lang and Rosen, 2002).

Lang *et al.* (2006) conducted another similarly designed randomized controlled study on hypnosis in 236 women undergoing large-core breast biopsies. Large-core breast biopsy is known to be highly anxiety provoking (Bugbee *et al.*, 2005) and was chosen as a representative model for outpatient surgery performed under local anesthesia only. In all three conditions – standard care, structured empathy and self-hypnosis – pain increased linearly with procedure time. Both empathy and hypnosis interventions reduced pain perception, but only hypnosis had a significant beneficial impact on anxiety: patients' anxiety significantly heightened in the standard care group, remained unchanged in the structured empathy group, and declined significantly in the hypnosis group.

Based on these findings and the review of the literature, Flory *et al.* (2007, in press) concluded that:

> . . . there is overwhelming evidence for the effectiveness of hypnosis to reduce acute distress and pain during procedures. There is also support that hypnotic techniques can ameliorate the effects of analgesia and anesthesia, stabilize vital signs, reduce complications, facilitate healing and recovery, and overall reduce health care costs. Hypnosis, as an established valuable tool, is now ready for implementation into health care on a large scale.

APPLICATION OF HYPNOSIS IN PSYCHIATRY

Although hypnosis has been utilized as a psychiatric treatment since the time of ancient Greece (Maldonado and Spiegel, 2003), from the eighteenth century it evolved intimately with psychiatry. As mentioned earlier, Mesmer's magnetic theory of illness and treatment was discredited by the French investigating commission. The commission concluded that the clinical improvements seen in Mesmer's patients were due to the phenomenon of suggestions. This led Ellenberger (1970), a well-known historian of dynamic psychiatry, to credit Mesmer as the father of formal psychotherapy, because he was the first physician to conceptualize the talking interaction between a doctor and a patient as a form of formal treatment. Lopez (1993) believes most of the conditions treated by Mesmer were psychiatric conditions that nowadays would be labelled psychosomatic or somatoform disorders. It would appear that Mesmer not only found an alternative method of treatment – talk therapy or psychotherapy – but also forged the link between hypnosis (the power of suggestions) and psychiatry.

In the 19th century the association between psychiatry and hypnosis was further solidified. In the later part of the 18th century psychiatry was fascinated with the understanding and treatment of dissociative disorders, mainly conversion and somatoform disorders. Jean Charcot and Pierre Janet, two distinguished neurologists from France, became very interested in psychiatry, especially for the treatment of conversion disorders. Both developed an international reputation by successfully treating these conditions with hypnosis. Moreover, Charcot and Janet demonstrated that conversion symptoms could be produced by hypnosis. What was remarkable about this approach was the fact that these physicians were able to develop experimental models of psychopathology. Physicians from all over the world, including Breuer and Freud, visited Charcot's and Janet's clinics to learn about hypnotherapy.

Although Freud abandoned hypnosis later, he published *Studies in Hysteria* (Breuer and Freud, 1893–95/1955) jointly with Breuer. The pair used hypnotic age regression to treat hysterical symptoms and developed the unconscious theory of conscious symptoms. They theorized that the 'hypnoid' states, although they can be normal, at times can be mobilized to resolve unconscious conflicts, thus 'serving as building blocks of hysterical symptomatology' (Maldonado and Spiegel, 2003, p. 1286). Unfortunately, both Charcot and Janet erroneously believed that dissociation was a psychopathological state. As discussed in Chapter 1, Hilgard (1977) considers dissociation to be a normal cognitive process that can range from mild to extreme dissociation (it can be normal or abnormal – a question of degree), and hence he called his theory of hypnosis the neodissociation theory.

After its rejection by Freud, hypnosis remained latent for almost a decade. However, in the 20th century interest in the application of hypnosis to psychiatry was revived during World War II. Army psychiatrists found hypnosis to be effective in the treatment of 'traumatic neurosis', which nowadays we would call post-traumatic stress disorder. The later part of the twentieth century saw intensive laboratory investigations of the hypnotic phenomenon, ranging from:

> . . . studies of the relationships among hypnotizability, placebo response, and acupuncture to studies of the differential hypnotizability of patients with psychosis and other psychiatric disorders to investigations used in determining neurophysiological correlates of the hypnotic state and hypnotic capacity, all with varying success. (Maldonado and Spiegel, 2003, p. 1286)

From this review, it would appear that modern hypnosis had an intimate evolving relationship with psychiatry. Hypnosis provided both a model of psychopathology and a treatment intervention. It also provided Freud with the impetus to develop his unconscious theory of the mind. With the endorsement of hypnosis by the British Medical Association, the American Medical Association and the American Psychiatric Association, it became recognized as a legitimate therapeutic tool. It is therefore not surprising that hypnosis has been used as an adjunctive tool with a variety of psychiatric conditions, including anxiety, depression, dissociative disorders, somatoform disorders, eating disorders, sleep disorders and sexual disorders.

The following part of this chapter describes the application of hypnosis to five well-known psychiatric conditions: anxiety disorders, post-traumatic stress disorder, dissociative disorders, conversion disorders and insomnia. Chapter 5 describes in detail the hypnotic treatment protocol for treating clinical depression.

Anxiety disorders

With the exception of substance abuse disorders, anxiety disorders are the most common psychiatric problem treated by psychiatrists and psychotherapists in Western societies. They are also comorbid with various medical and psychiatric conditions. Anxiety disorders are characterized by three categories of symptoms: physiological reactivity, maladaptive cognitions and avoidance behaviors.

Modern hypnotherapy combines hypnosis with cognitive behavior therapy (CBT) (Boutin and Tosi, 1983; Golden, 2006; Golden *et al.*, 1987) in the management of anxiety disorders. This approach is referred to as *cognitive-behavioral hypnotherapy* (CBH). Kirsch *et al.* (1995) from their meta-analysis of 18 studies in which CBT was compared to CBH (the same CBT treatment with hypnosis added) concluded that hypnosis enhances the effectiveness of CBT. Boutin and Tosi (1983) found that rational directed hypnotherapy, which is a form of CBH, was more effective than hypnosis alone in the treatment of test anxiety. Similarly, Gibbons *et al.* (1970) found hypnosis to enhance the effect of systematic desensitization.

There are three ways in which hypnotherapy, as an adjunct to CBT, can reduce symptoms of anxiety. First, hypnosis can be used to reduce the physiological reactivity associated with anxiety disorders. This can be achieved by inducing deep relaxation and teaching the anxious patient to 'let go' via self-hypnosis. Hypnosis also provides a modality for creating anti-anxiety feelings such as floating away in a tranquil setting (Spiegel and Spiegel, and Stanton, in Hammond, 1990, pp. 157–9) or feeling distant from tension-producing sensation (Finkelstein, 1990). These procedures provide the patient with the confidence to control anxiety feelings and sensations.

Second, hypnosis can solidify cognitive restructuring produced by CBT by focusing on negative self-hypnosis (NSH). Anxious patients have the tendency to ruminate with self-defeating and negative thoughts. Araoz (1981) has pointed out that this process is a form of NSH. CBH is particularly useful for overcoming NSH because hypnosis creates positive feelings, increases self-esteem (via ego-strengthening), and fosters a sense of perceived-self-efficacy (ability to let go) and a sense of self-control.

Third, hypnosis provides a powerful tool for dealing with avoidance behaviors. Because hypnosis can produce significant physiological, somatic and perceptual changes, it provides a powerful context for flooding and systematic desensitization procedures. As mentioned before, Gibbons *et al.* (1970) found hypnosis enhanced the effect of systematic desensitization. The split screen technique (a modified version of the screen technique described by Spiegel and Spiegel, 2004, p. 279) has also been found to be effective in dealing with fearful situations and avoidance behaviors.

The split screen technique consists of the following components:

○ hypnotic induction

○ deepening

○ intensifying positive feeling

○ intensifying the 'adult ego' state.

The person is asked to imagine sitting in front of a large split screen (left and right). They are then asked to project their adult ego state to the right side of the screen, and to project their anxious part to the left side of the screen. They then imagine the ego from the right side helping the left side, and integrate the two parts. According to Spiegel and Spiegel (2004, p. 279), the split screen technique:

> . . . teaches patients how to face and deal with stressors that complicate their anxiety while controlling their somatic response. It frees them to use focused concentration to expand their repertoire of responses, thereby feeling less helpless in the face of anxiety.

Hypnosis can also be used for recovering and restructuring unconscious factors underlying the anxiety disorder. However, within the modern hypnotherapy framework, uncovering unconscious materials is normally carried out only when the anxious patient does not respond to the usual CBH and the therapist has already worked on resistance issues and believes that some additional leverage is necessary. Golden *et al.* (1987, p. 272) use the following instruction with their hypnotized subjects to access unconscious information:

ACCESSING UNCONSCIOUS INFORMATION

And, as you already know, you are able to remember things when you are in a trance that you have repressed . . . memories, events, feelings, that are related to your problem . . . And you can tell me about them now . . . as you remember them.

Post-traumatic stress disorder (PTSD)

From their comprehensive review of the literature on hypnosis for the treatment of post-traumatic conditions, Cardeña *et al.* (2000) concluded that there are compelling reasons and clinical observations to recommend the use of hypnosis as an adjunct for the treatment of PTSD. They go on to say that hypnotic procedures can serve as a useful adjunct to cognitive, exposure and psychodynamic therapies. This recommendation is reinforced by the fact that patients with post-traumatic conditions seem to be more hypnotically suggestible than most other patient populations (Bryant *et al.*, 2001; Spiegel *et al.*, 1988; Stutman and Bliss, 1985).

However, Maldonado and Spiegel (2003) do point out that successful psychotherapy with PTSD requires a multimodal approach consisting of cognitive restructuring, emotional expression and relationship management. With this caveat, Spiegel (1993) utilizes hypnosis with PTSD as an adjunct to psychotherapy, which can be summarized in eight principles (the 8Cs): confrontation, confession, consolation, condensation, consciousness, concentration, control and congruence. These are briefly described below.

Confrontation

It is important to confront the traumatic events directly rather than attributing the symptoms to some personality traits. A careful history is therefore taken to determine the relationship between the traumatic events and the development of the PTSD symptoms. Many patients attempt to suppress the traumatic experience because it may be too upsetting for them or to their close contacts. For these patients to overcome their symptoms, it will be important for them to admit the damage caused by the trauma and consequently confront the trauma.

Confession

It is often necessary for the patients to confess their feelings and experiences to the therapist, even though they may be shameful and embarrassing. When traumatized, victims are subjected to a variety of experiences, including feeling helpless, degraded, frightened, or acting contrary to their beliefs and values. Such experiences can induce profound shame, guilt and embarrassment, and some trauma survivors even go beyond 'survivor guilt' and begin to believe their identity is spoilt and they can never be the same person again.

In the case formulation described in Chapter 2 (Appendix 2B), because Cathy was subjected to emotional and physical abuse from her alcoholic husband, she believes 'I am no one', 'I have no confidence', 'He destroyed me; he took away my pride and my dignity' and 'He turned me into a failure; he took away my personality'. In therapy it is necessary to encourage PTSD patients to confess their deeds and emotions, however embarrassing or repugnant they may be. From the details provided by the patient, the therapist is able to help the patient distinguish between misplaced guilt and remorse.

Consolation

It is very important for therapists to be sensitive, consoling, empathic and non-judgemental when patients express their intense emotions and experiences related to the trauma, otherwise the patients will feel victimized once again. During trauma work, it is very easy for a kind of traumatic transference to develop between the patient and therapist, whereby the patient feels victimized. For example, when 'working through' with a rape victim, the patient may feel as if he or she is re-victimized by the therapist. The use of hypnosis does not prevent the development of such transference reaction. In fact, hypnosis, because of its ability to intensify experience, can elicit such a reaction earlier than in regular therapy. Regular exploration with the patient to find whether the therapy is useful or harmful can prevent the development of the transference reaction and convey to the patient that the therapist is concerned, and this will allow the patient to differentiate the therapy from the trauma.

Condensation

When working through traumatic memories it is unnecessary to review every detail of the experience. It is sufficient to find out which aspects of the trauma were the critical elements that make it upsetting to the patient. This can be achieved by asking the patient, 'What was the worst part of it for you?' From the account, the therapist can identify the image that condenses a crucial aspect of the traumatic experience. Focusing on the condensed representation of the trauma reduces the overwhelming feelings associated with the whole context of the trauma and allows the therapist to work with a concrete aspect of the trauma.

Consciousness

One of the major goals of psychotherapy with PTSD patients is to bring to conscious awareness previously repressed memories. Bringing traumatic memories into consciousness gives the patient the opportunity to acknowledge and deal with them. Various hypnotic techniques such as age regression and the split screen technique can be used to bring repressed traumatic memories into consciousness.

Concentration

Focused concentration allows the patient to work on specific experiences and memories of the trauma, rather than being flooded by the whole array of memories and negative associations and adverse implications. This focused approach to therapy makes the accessing and restructuring of the memories and affect more manageable to the patient. Often trauma patients fear they will lose control and become defenceless once they allow themselves to remember the details of the trauma. The focused concentration approach dispels such fears and provides confidence to the patients to explore other aspects of their trauma and work on specific goals. Concentration and focused attention are highly intensified by hypnosis. From the structured and intensified experience of the hypnotic trance, 'patients learn that they can think about the traumatic experience in a constructive and controlled fashion rather than trying not to think about it' and the 'implied message is that once the therapeutic process is over, the patient will then be freer to attend to other things' (Spiegel and Spiegel, 2004, p. 436).

Control

The main goal of psychotherapy is to give the patient a sense of control. One of the most distressing aspects of severe trauma is the sense of loss of control. Patients feel they no longer have control over their physical and emotional experience, which in turn causes a sense of helplessness and hopelessness. It is therefore very important for the therapist to conduct psychotherapy in such a way that the patient feels empowered. Hypnosis provides a powerful context for teaching patients how to master past experiences and current symptoms (e.g. flashbacks, anxiety, nightmares) and the acquired sense of control can be solidified by teaching patients self-hypnosis. The therapist can also reinforce the notion that:

> . . . hypnosis is a collaborative enterprise, not something done to the patient by the therapist, and that hypnosis is also a self-hypnotic tool available to patients at any time to enable them to help themselves better cope with the aftermath of trauma (Spiegel and Spiegel, 2004, p. 436).

Congruence

Another important goal of psychotherapy with PTSD patients is to help them integrate dissociated or repressed traumatic material in such a way that they can tolerate experiencing the memories while staying grounded in the present. Hypnotic strategies such as reframing, rewriting the past, and the split screen technique provide a useful tool for separating the past from the present.

Dissociative disorders

Hypnosis has been found to be an effective adjunctive tool in the treatment of dissociative disorders. Dissociative disorders (dissociative amnesia, dissociative fugue, dissociative identity disorder, and depersonalization) are characterized by changes in a person's sense of identity, memory or consciousness (American Psychiatric Association, 2000), and they all involve varying degrees of dissociation. Since dissociation is one of the main components of hypnosis, it makes sense to utilize hypnosis in identifying and controlling the dissociative symptoms (Kluft, 1993; Spiegel and Spiegel, 2004).

Because dissociative disorders often affect intra-psychic, interpersonal and memory functioning, many pre-existing problems are magnified. Hypnosis is helpful both in clarifying diagnosis and facilitating psychotherapy. For example, hypnotic induction in a dissociative identity disorder patient can be easily utilized to switch identity. Such an incident provides very useful diagnostic information. Dissociative symptoms can be deliberately induced either through age regression or having the patient re-experience the last time the dissociative symptoms occurred. In this structured way, the patient can be taught to bring on the symptom and thereby learn to control it. The following case example from Maldonado and Spiegel (2003, p. 1297) illustrates how hypnosis can be used in a structured manner to treat dissociative symptoms.

> A 16-year-old boy was brought to the emergency department writhing and screaming that he was possessed by 'demons of Satan'. He was initially diagnosed with schizophrenia and was given antipsychotic medication, to which he did not respond. His history indicated that he had been well until several months earlier, when his girlfriend had left him and he had made a suicide gesture in front of her home. She took him to the local pastor, who referred to the suicide attempt as 'Satan's work'. The boy then began having possession episodes in which he growled in a strange voice that threatened to put a curse on the patient and to transfer the curse to anyone who tried to interfere. The patient was amnesic for each episode afterward.
>
> The patient was examined with the HIP [Hypnotic Induction Profile] and scored 10 out of 10 points, indicating high hypnotizability. He was then age-regressed to the last possession episode, and he changed abruptly from being polite and subdued to harboring the delusional belief that he was possessed by a demon, laughing in a bizarre manner, sniffling, and growling. The regression was ended and he reassumed his more restrained demeanor. He was congratulated for having been able to bring on the possession episode. His parents were

encouraged not to panic as they had previously when these episodes occurred and also to change the bedroom arrangement in the home. He had been sharing a room with an older sister, who it turned out had been sexually active with her boyfriend. Within a few weeks the possession episodes stopped, and the patient maintained his improvement for years afterward without the use of antipsychotic medications.

Conversion disorders

As mentioned in Chapter 1, Charcot and Janet successfully treated a variety of conversion disorders with hypnosis. It is also well established that patients with conversion disorders have high hypnotic capacity. For example, Bliss (1984) found conversion patients to score an average of 9.7 on the Hypnotic Induction Profile (HIP) 12-point scale. This finding was corroborated by Maldonado (1996a, 1996b), which led him to hypothesize that patients with conversion disorder may be using their own capacity to dissociate to displace uncomfortable emotional feeling onto a chosen body part, which then becomes dysfunctional. Maldonado and Spiegel (2003) argue that since the hypnotic phenomena may be involved in the etiology of some conversion symptoms, hypnosis can be used to control the symptoms. Maldonado and Spiegel suggest that hypnosis can be used with conversion disorders in two ways: as a diagnostic tool, and as an adjunct to treatment.

Classical conversion disorders are more amenable to psychological manipulation, and this characteristic serves as very important diagnostic information. Conversely, when conversion disorders have some underlying organic causation or, when a bona fide medical condition is misdiagnosed as a conversion disorder, the symptoms are less malleable. Because hypnosis can bring on, worsen or ameliorate the conversion symptoms, it can be utilized as a diagnostic tool.

Hypnotic modulation of the conversion symptoms can also serve as a powerful therapeutic tool. Hypnotic modification and modulation of the symptoms help to convey to the patient that the symptoms are alien or threatening. The changes in symptom produced during or after the hypnotic induction can then be used constructively to demonstrate to the patient that the symptom can be controlled, and that the patient can learn to control the symptom via self-hypnosis.

Hypnosis can also be used to reduce the reactive anxiety associated with physical dysfunction or other conversion symptoms. Maldonado and Spiegel (2003) stress the importance of self-hypnosis in the management of the secondary symptoms. They also emphasize the importance of gradual rehabilitation rather than quick removal of the symptom. They caution against hypnotic elimination of a symptom without first understanding its meaning and purpose, and recommend three phases of treatment with conversion disorder.

In the first phase, the meaning of the symptom is explored. This allows the therapist a better understanding of the dynamics of the symptom(s). The second phase involves symptom alteration and extinction. Symptom alteration can be induced through either *symptom substitution*, in which a given symptom is exchanged for another symptom that is less impairing (e.g. perception of intense pain exchanged for numbness), or *symptom extinction*, in which a patient agrees to 'give up' the symptom after working through the problem with the therapist. The third phase involves maximizing the patient's level of functioning.

Insomnia

Because insomnia is a complex, multifaceted complaint that may involve difficulty falling asleep, staying asleep, early morning awakenings and/or a complaint of non-refreshing sleep that produces significant impairment (American Psychiatric Association, 2000), a multimodal approach to treatment is required. The two most common types of insomnia (not including insomnia associated with a medical disorder) are adjustment and psychophysiological sleep disorders.

Adjustment sleep disorder is a condition in which an individual has experienced a significant life stressor (such as death of a loved one or being diagnosed with a life-threatening illness) which interferes with sleep. This type of sleep disturbance is commonly transient and generally abates within a month. However, when this type of transient insomnia does not attenuate, it can progress to chronic insomnia, often accompanied by depression. In comparison, *psychophysiological insomnia* results from the presence of heightened arousal in which somatized tension and learned sleep preventing associations (e.g. nervousness, anxiety, ruminative thoughts) interfere with nocturnal sleep.

Hypnosis can be a very useful component of treatment, particularly as a powerful tool for reducing the heightened psychophysiological arousal and as a vehicle for exploring and restructuring unconscious conflicts (in the event that the patient is not responding to regular therapy and the patient or therapist suspects unconscious etiology). Hypnosis as a single treatment modality has been used successfully to alleviate insomnia (Dement and Vaughan, 2000; Hadley, 1996; Hammond, 1990; Hauri, 1993, 2000; Kryger, 2004; Spiegel and Spiegel, 1990; Stanton, 1990, 1999; Weaver and Becker, 1996). Hypnosis and self-hypnosis both offer rapid methods to manage anxiety and worry, facilitating deep relaxation, and controlling mental overactivity and decreasing physiological arousal, which are cardinal symptoms of insomnia (Bauer and McCanne, 1980; Hammond, 1990). Self-hypnosis is considered a voluntary relaxation technique (Dement and Vaughan, 2000) that is similar to meditation because it can ease the body and mind, preparing the body for sleep (Kryger, 2004).

Several other types of sleep disorders, including hypersomnias, circadian rhythm disorders and parasomnias, have been successfully treated using hypnosis as either a single- or multi-treatment modality (Graci and Hardie, 2007). It should be noted that these sleep disorders result from biological factors and may not be amenable to hypnotic interventions. However, if psychological and/or behavioral issues are contributing factors, then hypnotherapy may be effective in reducing arousal states. Cognitive-behavioral techniques have been found to be the 'gold standard' in maintaining long-term treatment gains.

Clinical hypnosis is a safe and effective method of treating insomnia because it allows the clinician to gain access to the underlying problem (Modlin, 2002). Several trials as well as several reviews (Lichstein and Riedel, 1994; Morin, 1999; Morin et al., 1999) and meta-analyses (Morin et al., 1994; Murtagh and Greenwood, 1995) have examined the efficacy of relaxation and hypnosis for the treatment of insomnia (Morin, 1999). A 1994 meta-analysis of 59 studies (Morin et al., 1994) reported that psychological interventions averaging five hours produced reliable changes in sleep onset and time spent awake after an awakening. A 1996 National Institutes of Health consensus panel concluded that hypnosis and biofeedback produced significant changes in some aspects of sleep. However, it was unclear whether the magnitude of improvements in sleep onset and total sleep time were clinically significant (National Institutes of Health, 1996).

It is not surprising that studies have yielded conflicting findings. Clinicians trained in hypnotherapy should consult with a sleep professional when designing studies to ensure that the population is homogeneous in terms of sleep disturbance. As discussed earlier, somatically based insomnias have not been amenable to hypnotic interventions (Weitzenhoffer, 2000). In contrast, some psychological insomnias (i.e. precipitated by upset either prior to sleep onset or waking up after sleep onset and experiencing difficulty returning to sleep because of anxiety about not sleeping or losing sleep) are very amenable to hypnosis.

Relaxation training and hypnosis can be effective in the treatment of late-life insomnia (Morin *et al.*, 1999). A randomized trial found that cognitive-behavioral therapy (alone and in combination with pharmacological therapy) was effective in reducing time awake after sleep onset in elderly patients (Morin *et al.*, 1999). Whereas drug therapy alone was more effective than placebo, only those patients using the behavioral approach maintained treatment gains at follow-up. Although pharmacological treatments produced somewhat faster sleep improvements in the short term, behavioral approaches, including hypnosis and relaxation training, showed comparable effects in the intermediate term (four to eight weeks). In the long term (six to twenty-four months), behavioral approaches, including hypnosis and relaxation training, showed more favorable outcomes than drug therapies (Morin *et al.*, 1994).

Graci and Sexton-Radek (2006) have developed a comprehensive psychological approach, combining CBT with hypnosis, for the treatment of insomnia. This is an eight-week treatment program consisting of formal assessment, psychoeducation, sleep hygiene, CBT, hypnosis, and strategies for relapse prevention. The hypnosis component involves induction of relaxation, imagery training, and self-hypnosis aided by CD or cassette tape of hypnosis. The following script from Graci and Hardie (2007, in press) illustrates the kinds of hypnotic suggestions that can be utilized with insomnia.

USING HYPNOTIC SUGGESTION WITH INSOMNIA

I want you to imagine walking towards your bedroom, and as you are walking you are giving yourself permission to leave all worries, concerns or anything that is troubling you outside of your bedroom. When you awaken in the morning, you can retrieve these worries, concerns or troubles when you walk out of your bedroom. There is no need to bring these with you because your bedroom is a safe haven. It is your personal safety zone. It is here that you can experience comfort, safety and peace.

You notice the bedroom door is getting closer and closer and you are feeling more and more relaxed and peaceful. There is nothing of concern to you as you approach your bedroom, and this feeling of relaxation becomes deeper and deeper, especially as you walk into your bedroom. You notice that you are feeling calmer, more secure, and more peaceful as you approach your bed. Your limbs are growing heavier and heavier as you pull back the covers of your bed. As you get into bed, you notice how comfortable you are lying in your bed. Your mind is quiet and you feel calm and relaxed. Your eyelids are beginning to get heavier and heavier and you welcome this feeling.

When you are ready, your eyelids close. You are lying in comfort and you notice that you are free of any emotional or physical discomfort. You don't have any concerns because your mind is very quiet and calm. You are feeling sleepier and sleepier. There is no need to check the clock because your body knows how to fall asleep, how to stay asleep and how to wake up when it is ready to awaken. The clock is unimportant and you will not feel a need to look at it because you are working with your body – nature's original sleep/wake clock. It is important to remember that when your body is ready to sleep, it will sleep. This experience of sleep will be a deep and profound sleep. If you wake up during the night, you will easily return to sleep even if you have gotten up to use the bathroom, because your body knows how to sleep. You feel peaceful and safe and are very, very sleepy. You know that your body knows how to sleep because you have done it since you were a child. And much like a child, you welcome sleep and your body will wake up when it has had enough sleep. It is important to sleep just long enough and to keep the same bedtimes and wake times, even during the weekends. Rest assured that you will sleep well. You have the ability to experience deep restorative sleep, just as you have the ability to manage the day-to-day activities of your life right now. When you wake to your alarm in the morning, you will feel refreshed and energetic and ready to start your day.

Although psychological treatment for insomnia is initially more time-consuming and more expensive than hypnotic medication, there are long-lasting benefits associated with psychological interventions. For instance, over the course of total physician visits and prescriptions, it may be more cost effective for patients to engage in behavioral treatments (Graci and Sexton-Radek, 2006). Current research findings support the use of psychological approaches for treating 'non-biologic' sleep disorders such as insomnia because these approaches target and resolve the underlying problem(s) associated with sleep disturbance, whereas pharmaceutical agents are a 'band-aid' approach to treatment. Because of its ability to produce deep relaxation, hypnosis should be routinely used as an adjunct to the multimodal therapy of insomnia. However, further empirical research is required to demonstrate the additive effect of hypnosis to the multimodal treatment of insomnia.

REFERENCES

American Psychiatric Association (2000). *Diagnostic and Statistical Manual of Mental Disorders*. 4th ed., text rev. Washington, DC: American Psychiatric Association.

Araoz DL. (1981). Negative self-hypnosis. *Journal of Contemporary Psychotherapy* 12: 45–52.

Barabasz A, Watkins JG. (2005). *Hypnotherapeutic Techniques*. 2nd ed. New York: Brunner-Routledge.

Bauer KE, McCanne TR. (1980). An hypnotic technique for treating insomnia. *International Journal of Clinical and Experimental Hypnosis* 28: 1–5.

Bliss EL. (1984). Hysteria and hypnosis. *Journal of Nervous and Mental Disorders* 172: 203–6.

Boutin GE, Tosi DJ. (1983). Modification of irrational ideas and test anxiety through rational stage directed hypnotherapy RSDH. *Journal of Clinical Psychology* 39: 382–91.

Breuer J, Freud S. (1893–95/1955). In Strachey J, editor. *The Standard Edition of the Complete Works of Sigmund Freud, Vol. 2*. London: Hogarth.

Brown D. (2007). Evidence-based hypnotherapy for asthma: a critical review. *International Journal of Clinical and Experimental Hypnosis* 55: 220–49.

Brown PD, Fromm E. (1986). *Hypnosis and Behavioral Medicine*. Hillsdale, NJ: Erlbaum.

Bryant RA, Guthrie RM, Moulds ML. (2001). Hypnotizability is acute stress disorder. *American Journal of Psychiatry* 158: 600–4.

Bryant R, Moulds M, Gutherie R, *et al.* (2005). The additive benefit of hypnosis and cognitive-behavioral therapy in treating acute stress disorder. *Journal of Consulting and Clinical Psychology* 73: 334–40.

Bugbee ME, Wellisch DK, Arnott IM, *et al.* (2005). Breast core-needle biopsy: clinical trial of relaxation technique versus medication versus no intervention for anxiety reduction. *Radiology* 234: 73–8.

Cardeña E, Maldonado J, Van der Hart O, *et al.* (2000). Hypnosis. In: Foa EB, Keane TM, Friedman MJ, editors. *Effective Treatments for PTSD* (pp. 247–79). New York: Guilford Press.

Chambless DL, Hollon SD. (1998). Defining empirically-supported therapies. *Journal of Consulting and Clinical Psychology* 66: 7–18.

Conn JH. (1957). Historical aspects of scientific hypnosis. *Journal of Clinical and Experimental Hypnosis* 5: 127–34.

Covino NA, Frankel FH. (1993). Hypnosis and relaxation in the medically ill. *Psychotherapy and Psychosomatics* 60: 75–90.

Dement W, Vaughan C. (2000). *The Promise of Sleep*. New York: Random House, Inc.

Elkins G, Jensen M, Patterson DR. (2007). Hypnotherapy for the management of chronic pain. *International Journal of Clinical and Experimental Hypnosis* 55: 275–87.

Ellenberger H. (1970). *Discovery of the Unconscious: the history and evolution of dynamic psychiatry.* New York: Basic Books.

Elliotson J. (1943). *Numerous Cases of Surgical Operations Without Pain in the Mesmeric State.* London: Bailliere.

Esdaile J. (1846/1976). *Mesmerism in India and its Practical Application in Surgery and Medicine.* London: Longman, Brown, Green and Longmans. Reprinted New York: Arno Press.

Finkelstein S. (1990). The private refuge. In: Hammond DC, editor. *Handbook of Hypnotic Suggestions and Metaphors.* New York: WW Norton and Company, Inc.

Flory N, Salazar GM, Lang EV. (2007). Hypnosis for acute distress management during medical procedures. *International Journal of Clinical and Experimental Hypnosis* 55: 303–17.

Gibbons D, Kilbourne L, Saunders A, *et al.* (1970). The cognitive control of behavior: a comparison of systematic desensitization and hypnotically-induced 'direct experience' techniques. *American Journal of Clinical Hypnosis* 12: 141–5.

Gibson HB, Heap M. (1991). *Hypnosis in Therapy.* Hove, East Sussex: Lawrence Erlbaum Associates Ltd., Publishers.

Golden WL. (1994). Cognitive-behavioral hypnotherapy for anxiety. *Journal of Cognitive Psychotherapy: An International Quarterly* 8(4): 265–74.

Golden WL. (2006). Hypnotherapy for anxiety, phobias, and psychophysiological disorders. In: Chapman R, editor. *The Clinical Use of Hypnosis with Cognitive Behavior Therapy: a practitioner's casebook.* New York: Springer Publishing Company.

Golden WL, Dowd ET, Friedberg F. (1987). *Hypnotherapy: a modern approach.* New York: Pergamon Press.

Graci G, Hardie JC. (2007). Evidence-based hypnotherapy for the management of sleep disorders. *International Journal of Clinical and Experimental Hypnosis* 55: 288–302.

Graci G, Sexton-Radek K. (2006). Treating sleep disorders using cognitive behavioral therapy and hypnosis. In: Chapman RH, editor. *The Clinical Use of Hypnosis in Cognitive Behavior Therapy: a practitioner's casebook* (pp. 295–331). New York: Springer Publishing Company.

Hadley J. (1996). Sleep. In: Hadley J, Staudacher C, editors. *Hypnosis for Change.* New York: MJF Books.

Hammond DC, editor. (1990). *Handbook of Hypnotic Suggestions and Metaphors.* New York: Norton.

Hammond DC. (2007). Review of the efficacy of clinical hypnosis with headaches and migraines. *International Journal of Clinical and Experimental Hypnosis* 55: 207–19.

Hauri PJ. (1993). Consulting about insomnia: a method and some preliminary data. *Journal of Sleep Research and Sleep Medicine* 16: 344–50.

Hauri PJ. (2000). The many faces of insomnia. In: Mostofsky DI, Barlow DH, editors. *The Management of Stress and Anxiety in Medical Disorders* (pp. 143–59). Needham Heights, MA: Allyn and Bacon.

Hartland J. (1971). *Medical and Dental Hypnosis and its Clinical Applications.* 2nd ed. London: Bailliere Tindall.

Hawkins PJ. (2006). *Hypnosis and Stress: a guide for clinicians.* Chichester, West Sussex: John Wiley and Sons, Ltd.

Hilgard ER. (1977). *Divided Consciousness: multiple controls in human thought and action.* New York: John Wiley and Sons.

Katon W, Roy-Byrne, Russo J, *et al.* (2002). Cost-effectiveness and cost off-set of a collaborative care intervention for primary care patients with panic disorder. *Archives of General Psychiatry* 59: 1098–104.

Kirsch I, Montgomery G, Sapirstein G. (1995). Hypnosis as an adjunct to cognitive-behavioral psychotherapy: a meta-analysis. *Journal of Consulting and Clinical Psychology* 63: 214–20.

Kluft RP. (1993). The treatment of dissociative disorder patients: an overview of discoveries, successes and failures. *Dissociation* 7: 135–7.

Kogan M, Biswas A, Spiegel D. (1997). Effect of medical and psychotherapeutic treatment on the survival of women with metastatic breast carcinoma. *Cancer* 80: 225–30.

Kryger M. (2004). *A Woman's Guide to Sleep Disorders.* New York: McGraw-Hill.

Lang EV, Benotsch EG, Fick LJ, *et al.* (2000). Adjunctive non-pharmacologic analgesia for invasive medical procedures: a randomized trial. *Lancet* 355: 1486–90.

Lang EV, Berbaum KS, Faintuch S, *et al.* (2006). Adjunctive self-hypnotic relaxation for outpatient medical procedures: a prospective randomized trial with women undergoing large core breast biopsy. *Pain* 126: 165–74.

Lang EV, Chen F, Fick LJ, *et al.* (1998). Determinants of intravenous conscious sedation for arteriography. *Journal of Vascular and Interventional Radiology* 9: 407–12.

Lang EV, Hatsiopoulou O, Koch T, *et al.* (2005). Can words hurt?: patient-provider interactions during invasive procedures. *Pain* 114(1–2): 303–9.

Lang EV, Joyce JS, Spiegel D, *et al.* (1996). Self-hypnotic relaxation during interventional radiological procedures: effects on pain perception and intravenous drug use. *International Journal of Experimental and Clinical Hypnosis* 44: 106–19.

Lang EV, Lutgendorf S, Logan H, *et al.* (1999). Nonpharmacologic analgesia and anxiolysis for interventional radiological procedures. *Seminars in Interventional Radiology* 16: 113–23.

Lang EV, Rosen M. (2002). Cost analysis of adjunct hypnosis for sedation during outpatient interventional procedures. *Radiology* 222: 375–82.

Levitan AA, Harbaugh TE. (1992). Hypnotizability and hypnoanalgesia: hypnotizability of patients using hypnoanalgesia during surgery. *American Journal of Clinical Hypnosis* 34: 223–6.

Lichstein KL, Riedel BW. (1994). Behavioral assessment and treatment of insomnia: a review with an emphasis on clinical application. *Behavioral Therapy* 25: 659–88.

Lopez CA. (1993). Franklin and Mesmer: an encounter. *Yale Journal of Biological Medicine* 66: 325–31.

Lynn SJ, Kirsch I, Barabasz A, *et al.* (2000). Hypnosis as an empirically supported clinical intervention: the state of the evidence and a look to the future. *International Journal of Clinical and Experimental Hypnosis* 48: 239–58.

Maldonado JR. (1996a). *Physiological Correlates of Conversion Disorders.* Paper presented at the 149th annual meeting of the American Psychiatric Association, New York.

Maldonado JR. (1996b). *Psychological and Physiological Factors in the Production of Conversion Disorder.* Paper presented at the Society for Clinical and Experimental Hypnosis annual meeting, Tampa, Florida.

Maldonado JR, Spiegel D. (2003). Hypnosis. In: Hales RE, Yudofsky SC, editors. *Textbook of Psychiatry.* 4th ed (pp. 1285–331). American Psychiatric Association: Washington, DC.

Modlin T. (2002). Sleep disorders and hypnosis: to cope or cure? *Sleep and Hypnosis* 4: 39–46.

Montgomery GH, DuHamel KN, Redd WH. (2000). A meta-analysis of hypnotically induced analgesia: how effective is hypnosis? *International Journal of Clinical and Experimental Hypnosis* 48(2): 138–53.

Morin CM. (1999). Empirically supported psychological treatments: a natural extension of the scientist-practitioner paradigm. *Canadian Psychology* 40: 312–15.

Morin CM, Culbert JP, Schwartz SM. (1994). Nonpharmacological interventions for insomnia: a meta-analysis of treatment efficacy. *American Journal of Psychiatry* 151: 1172–80.

Morin CM, Mimeault V, Gagne A. (1999). Nonpharmacological treatment of late-life insomnia. *Journal of Psychosomatic Research* 46:103–16.

Murtagh DR, Greenwood KM. (1995). Identifying effective psychological treatments for insomnia: a meta-analysis. *Journal of Consulting and Clinical Psychology* 63: 19–89.

National Institutes of Health. (1996). Technology Assessment Panel on Integration of Behavioral and Relaxation Approaches into the Treatment of Chronic Pain and Insomnia. *Journal of the American Medical Association* 276: 313–18.

Patterson DR, Jensen MP. (2003). Hypnosis and clinical pain. *Psychological Bulletin* 129: 495–521.

Pinnell CA, Covino NA. (2000). Empirical findings on the use of hypnosis in medicine: a critical review. *International Journal of Clinical and Experimental Hypnosis* 48: 170–94.

Rosenberg S. (1982–83). Hypnosis in cancer care: imagery to enhance the control of physiological and psychological 'side-effects' of cancer therapy. *American Journal of Clinical Hypnosis* 25: 122–7.

Ruzyla-Smith P, Barabasz A, Barabasz M, *et al.* (1995). Effects of hypnosis on the immune response: B-cells, T-cells, helper and suppressor cells. *American Journal of Clinical Hypnosis* 38: 71–9.

Spiegel, D. (1993). Hypnosis in the treatment of posttraumatic stress disorders. In: Rhue JW, Lynn SJ, Kirsch I, editors. *Handbook of Clinical Hypnosis* (pp. 493–508). Washington, DC: American Psychological Association.

Spiegel D, Hunt T, Dondershine HE. (1988). Dissociation and hypnotizability in posttraumatic stress disorder. *American Journal of Psychiatry* 145: 301–5.

Spiegel D, Spiegel H. (1987). Forensic uses of hypnosis. In: Weiner IB, Hess AK, editors. *Handbook of Forensic Psychology* (pp. 490–507). New York: John Wiley and Sons.

Spiegel D, Spiegel H. (1990). Hypnosis techniques with insomnia. In: Hammond DC, editor. *Handbook of Hypnotic Suggestions and Metaphors* (p. 255). New York: WW Norton and Company, Inc.

Spiegel H, Spiegel D. (2004). *Trance and Treatment: clinical uses of hypnosis.* 2nd ed. Washington, DC: American Psychiatric Publishing, Inc.

Stanton H. (1990). Visualization for treating insomnia. In: Hammond DC, editor. *Handbook of Hypnotic Suggestions and Metaphors* (pp. 254–5). New York: WW Norton and Company, Inc.

Stanton HE. (1999). Hypnotic relaxation and insomnia: a simple solution? *Sleep and Hypnosis* 1: 64–7.

Stutman RK, Bliss EL. (1985). Posttraumatic stress disorder, hypnotizability, and imagery. *American Journal of Psychiatry* 142: 741–3.

Wain H. (1980). Pain control through the use of hypnosis. *American Journal of Clinical Hypnosis* 23: 41–6.

Weaver DB, Becker PM. (1996). *Treatment of Insomnia with Audiotaped Hypnosis.* 38th Annual Scientific Meeting and Workshops on Clinical Hypnosis. Orlando: American Society of Clinical Hypnosis.

Weitzenhoffer A. (2000). *The Practice of Hypnotism.* New York: John Wiley and Sons.

Whithead WE. (2006). Hypnosis for irritable bowel syndrome: the empirical evidence of therapeutic effects. *International Journal of Clinical and Experimental Hypnosis* 54: 7–20.

CHAPTER 4

Hypnotherapy with a Medical Condition: Migraine Headache

SUMMARY

This chapter reviews the theories and psychological treatment of migraine headache. The main focus is on the description of the hypnotherapy prototype for migraine. Eleven hypnotherapy components are described and illustrated by hypnotic suggestions scripts. Clinicians are encouraged to standardize these procedures and to validate the relative effectiveness of these procedures in the management of migraine.

INTRODUCTION

Migraine headache has been described in the medical literature from the time of Greco-Roman medicine, and it has since been the focus of considerable attention. Despite its long history and the various speculations about etiology and treatment, neither a comprehensive theory nor an effective treatment has yet been established. This chapter reviews the theories and the psychological treatment for migraine. The main focus is on the description of the hypnotherapy prototype for migraine.

DEFINITION AND DESCRIPTION

Migraine headaches are characterized by recurrent attacks of pain that vary widely in frequency, intensity and duration. The Headache Classification Committee of the International Headache Society: Second Edition (ICHD-II) (2004) lists 14 major categories of headaches. Migraine is listed as the first of the major categories, comprising migraine without aura, migraine with aura, and chronic migraine. Migraine attacks are associated with loss of appetite, nausea, vomiting and exaggerated sensitivity to light and sound, and often involve sensory, motor or mood disturbances. The *migraine with aura* is characterized by identifiable sensory disturbances that precede the head pain, whereas *migraine without aura* has a sudden onset and an intense throbbing, usually unilateral. *Chronic migraine* is diagnosed in patients having migraine on 15 days per month or more in the absence of medication overuse (Olesen and Lipton, 2006).

Some clinicians have questioned the validity of the categorial classification of headaches. For example, Bakal (1982) views chronic headache as falling on a continuum so that the differences between different types of headaches are quantitative rather then qualitative. According to this view, there are no separate categories of headache as such (e.g. migraine versus muscle contraction headache); instead, there is chronic headache, which varies among individuals in terms of its intensity and frequency. A key component of this model is that chronic experience of headache is itself a stressor for the patient, which may help to perpetuate the headache disorder. The chronic pain and distress associated with the headache thus add to the total psychological and physiological stress with which the patient must cope. Having chronic headaches thus renders the sufferer more susceptible to new headaches.

It is hypothesized by most writers (e.g. Dalessio, 1980) that the following physiological events occur during a migraine headache. During the pre-headache period there is an increased lability in the temporal artery, followed by vasoconstriction which may or may not be subjectively experienced or labelled as prodromal in nature. The most common prodromal signs include scotomata, hemianopia, unilateral paraesthesia and speech disorder. A rebound dilation phase involving the internal and external cranial arteries follows the constriction phase and is associated with the onset of headache. This phase is characterized by a subjective experience of throbbing and severe pain.

In the latter part of the headache period, edema of the vasculature occurs, causing abnormally large increases in the amount of fluid in the intercellular tissue space. This edema is accompanied by increased rigidity of the blood vessels. A steady aching pain, tenderness of the scalp, nausea, vomiting, dryness of the mouth, sweating and chills may distinguish the second phase (Dalessio, 1980). The post-headache phase is marked by pain from sustained contraction of the scalp and neck, which is accompanied by deep, aching pain. Recently it has been hypothesized that migraine may originate in the neurons in the brain stem (Holroyd, 2002).

Headaches are among the top 14 principal problems reported by outpatients attending office-based general practitioners (DeLozier and Gagnon, 1975). The annual prevalence rate of migraine is estimated to be 20 to 25% (Adams *et al.*, 1980). Although headaches involve no risk of mortality, approximately 20% of the cases are considered 'serious' or 'very serious' (Feuerstein and Gainer, 1982).

ETIOLOGY/CAUSES OF MIGRAINE

In discussing the etiology of migraine, Feuerstein and Gainer (1982) have emphasized the delineation of those factors that predispose an individual to headache from those that exacerbate and maintain it. These factors, they argue, may be quite different, and therefore their specification may help to clarify the controversies surrounding the various theories of migraine. The identification of predisposing, exacerbating and maintaining factors may also help to formulate appropriate treatment protocols.

Some of the factors that are assumed to predispose, maintain and/or worsen headaches include diet, weather, sleep, hormonal change, psychosocial stress and various medical disorders. These factors, however, only account for a small proportion of recurring headaches in that their removal often affords only modest benefits. Little research has been directed at the consequences of migraine, so even less attention has been paid to factors that maintain chronic headache. Similarly, there has been virtually no research on the relationship between efforts to manage or cope with stress in a naturalistic environment and the frequency and intensity of headache symptoms. However, a large body of research suggests that the way an individual copes with stress can influence not only physiological stress responses, but also the onset and course of symptoms (e.g. Holroyd and Andrasik, 1982). At this point it is not known what coping styles render individuals vulnerable to headache attacks.

Bakal (1982) has suggested an alternative approach to the study of the relationship between stress and headaches. Rather than studying the processes that mediate between the person and their environment, Bakal emphasizes exploring the relationship between the patient and their symptoms. Therefore the critical processes that mediate the chronic headache syndrome are found in the relationship among the symptoms experienced, the physiological mechanisms that mediate these symptoms and the cognitive evaluation of the condition as the disorder develops across time. Chronic headache, he suggests, should be viewed as a migraine pain disorder that is heavily influenced by the patient's cognitive actions and reactions in dealing with the symptoms themselves. At the behavioral level, a number of social learning factors such as pain behaviors, attention (secondary gain) for symptoms, pain medication and use of symptoms to avoid unpleasant environmental demands can prolong the occurrence of migraine (e.g. Philips, 1978).

The mechanisms that are considered of primary importance in the etiology of migraine are biological, psychological and psychophysiological. The biological theories focus on cerebrovascular mechanisms and emphasize the role of biochemical agents (e.g. serotonin, histamine and catecholamine) as links in the chain of events that lead to head pain. The psychological theories concentrate on the relationship between psychological variables (e.g. emotional specificity, psychodynamic factors, personality, stress, psychiatric conditions and reinforcements) and the predisposition to migraine. The psychophysiological theories emphasize the potential role of 'stress' in the etiology of migraine and attempt to elucidate the specific mechanisms by which stress could trigger a headache. While no single theory has been able to explain why certain individuals develop migraines and others do not, nor even why headaches develop in certain situations and not in others, recently many investigators have advocated integrating the above theories.

Two integrated models have been reported in the literature. The first is based on Wolff's studies of headaches (*see* Dalessio, 1980). Cinciripini *et al.*

(1981) noted that although earlier researchers acknowledged the importance of psychological factors in the etiology of migraine, they never elaborated on the possible psychological mechanism involved. They therefore attempted to specify the interactive roles of psychological and environmental factors in the pathophysiology of migraine. In encompassing environmental, physiological and psychological factors, and the current understanding of chronic pain, their model outlined the possible relationship between physiological, behavioral/environmental, and behavioral/cognitive variables that may be important in the development and maintenance of migraine headaches. Although the model seems to provide a comprehensive account of psychosocial factors in the development and maintenance of migraine, it does not specify the physiological reactions resulting from the interaction between biological and psychosocial/environmental factors.

The second model, while acknowledging the importance of psychological factors in the maintenance of migraine, emphasizes the central role of sympathetic activity. Mathew *et al.* (1982), in their sympathetic-adrenomedullary activation (SAA) model, hold that sympathetic adrenomedullary activation is involved in the causation of the prodromal vasoconstrictior phase of migraine. SAA forms an integral part of a non-specific stress response. A wide variety of stress-evoking situations (psychological, physical, environmental and biochemical) are associated with increased sympathetic activity and output of catecholamine, adrenaline and noradrenaline.

The SAA model regards chronic migraine sufferers as developing an over-sensitive cerebral vasculature to catecholamine, which in response to psychological stress (pleasant or unpleasant) and/or certain external or internal stimuli associated with arousal (e.g. exercise, orgasm, REM sleep, hypoglycemia, tyramine, phenylethylamine, amphetamine, nicotine, reserpine) leads to an increase in sympathetic tone, starting the first phase (vasoconstriction) of migraine. Mathew *et al.* (1982) provide several lines of evidence to show that relaxation-related therapies and most anti-migraine pharmacological agents relieve migraine by reducing sympathetic tone; i.e. they induce 'relaxation-related biochemical changes such as reduction in plasma catecholamine and platelet monoamine oxidase' (p. 16).

Although the SAA model emphasizes the central role of sympathetic activity, it seems to account for most of the psychological, physiological and environmental factors known to be associated with migraine. The model has two serious implications for migraine research and therapy. First, it regards psychological, physical and environmental factors as being independent of the over-sensitive vascular mechanism, though interactive. Second, according to the model, relaxation-related therapies and most anti-migraine drugs work by reducing sympathetic activity.

MANAGEMENT OF MIGRAINE

Although migraine has existed for centuries, there is as yet no truly adequate treatment for chronic migraine headache. Therefore it would be more accurate to speak of the management of migraine rather than its treatment. A variety of management techniques have been attempted with chronic migraine, ranging from surgery to psychotherapy. From his review of the pharmacological and psychological management of migraine, Alladin (1991) draws the following conclusions.

❍ Not all migraine sufferers benefit from pharmacotherapy. Pharmacological treatment can either be acute (abortive) or preventive (prophylactic). Acute treatment attempts to reverse or stop a headache's progression once it has started. Triptans have been successful in aborting migraine headache in about 20% to 68% of migraine patients (Taylor and Martin, 2004, p. 59). Preventive treatment is designed to reduce attack frequency and severity. Prophylactic medications for migraine are effective in reducing the frequency of attacks in less than 50% of the patients (Adelman *et al.*, 2002) and therefore Taylor and Martin (2004, p. 64) recommend that 'patients need to be told that a complete cure for headache is not possible with current migraine preventives and that it may take some time to see an improvement'. Mathew and Tfelt-Hansen (2006, p. 433) state 'Physicians should encourage the patient to develop realistic expectations of the treatment of chronic migraine. It is important to explain that migraine is a recurrent disorder and that there is no total cure; the best that can be done is to keep the headaches under some control with abortive as well as preventive medications.' Moreover, some of the medications that are effective in some respects have adverse side-effects and contraindications (Mathew and Tfelt-Hansen, 2006). For these reasons, there is a need for alternative treatment.

❍ The effectiveness of physical and surgical management of migraine is limited and unclear.

❍ Psychological procedures such as thermal and extracranial biofeedback, relaxation training, behavior therapy, cognitive therapy, and a combination of these procedures are generally effective in the management of migraine. Recently, a number of meta-analytic reviews indicated that relaxation training, temperature biofeedback training, temperature biofeedback plus relaxation training, EMG biofeedback training, cognitive-behavioral therapy (CBT), CBT plus temperature biofeedback are more effective than wait list and other controls (McGrath *et al.*, 2006). These behavioral interventions yielded 32% to 49% reductions in migraine versus 5% reduction for no-treatment controls. Moreover, the follow-up data (e.g. Blanchard *et al.*, 1997) showed that 91% of migraine headache sufferers remained significantly improved 5 years after completing behavioral headache treatment.

○ The effects of behavioral therapies are comparable to the effects of pharmacotherapy. Recent meta-analyses (*see* review by McGrath *et al.*, 2006) demonstrate virtually identical improvement in migraine when comparing propranolol, flunarizine, and combined relaxation with biofeedback training. These findings suggest that the 'best of the prophylactic medications and behavioral therapies may be equally viable treatment options' (McGrath *et al.*, 2006, p. 445).

HYPNOSIS IN THE MANAGEMENT OF MIGRAINE

A variety of hypnotic techniques has been used in the treatment of migraine. Hypnosis most often involves some form of relaxation in conjunction with hypnotic procedures designed to modify pain perception and/or the emotional state of the patient. Bakal (1982) views hypnosis as a cognitive tool for teaching patients how to minimize the pain during attacks and to become aware of psychological events that lead to headache attacks. Spanos *et al.* (1979) remark that the effectiveness or ineffectiveness of hypnosis and suggestion procedures in the control of pain is largely determined by the patient's ability or inability to generate pain-control cognitions. Post-hypnotic suggestions have also been used.

The general approach is ultimately directed at self-hypnosis, where the patient is able to implement specific strategies to reduce autonomic arousal, modify pain and enhance 'self-perception'. Specific techniques used with migraine include relaxation, glove anesthesia, and symptom transformation via imagery and ego-strengthening (Anderson *et al.*, 1975; Andreychuk and Skriver, 1975). Finer (1974) has suggested that hypnosis should be used as the first, rather than the last, line of treatment for migraine. Hammond (2007), from his recent review of the effectiveness of hypnotherapy with migraine, concludes that:

> . . . not only has hypnosis been shown to be efficacious with headache and migraine, but it is also a treatment that is relatively brief and cost effective. At the same time it has been found to be virtually free of the side effects, risks of adverse reactions, and the ongoing expense associated with the widely used medication treatments. Hypnosis should be recognized by the scientific, health care, and medical insurance communities as being an efficient evidence-based practice. (p. 216)

The National Institutes of Health Technology Assessment Panel on Integration of Behavioral and Relaxation Approaches into the Treatment of Chronic Pain and Insomnia (1996) also concluded, from a review of the outcome studies on hypnosis with pain, that hypnosis is effective with chronic pain, including headaches. Similarly, a meta-analysis review of contemporary research on hypnosis and pain management (Montgomery *et al.*, 2000) noted that hypnosis meets the American Psychological Association criteria (Chambless and Hollon, 1998) for being an efficacious and specific treatment for pain, showing superiority to medication, psychological placebos and other treatments. Finally, Hammond's (2007) review of the literature on the effectiveness of hypnosis in the treatment of headaches and migraines concluded that hypnotherapy meets the clinical psychology research criteria for being a well-established and efficacious treatment for tension and migraine headaches.

PROTOTYPE OF HYPNOTHERAPY FOR MIGRAINE

Guided by the findings from the psychological literature, I have adopted the following hypnotic procedure with migraine. This procedure targets the three main components of migraine:
1. physiological changes (usually blood vessel dilation)
2. the subjective experience of pain (aching, distress, fatigue, etc.)
3. behavior motivated by the pain (e.g. pill taking, withdrawal from family and social activities, absence from work).

The treatment prototype described below represents the routine hypnotic procedure I have been using over the past 20 years with migraine patients. Although the focus is on hypnotherapy, treatment usually involves a multimodal approach consisting of medication, cognitive behavior therapy, stress inoculation and pain management. It should also be borne in mind that migraine sufferers do not form a homogeneous group. The treatment should be adapted to each individual patient's clinical needs.

The hypnotherapy treatment prototype consists of 11 components:

- assessment and medical clearance
- education and establishment of rapport
- hypnotic induction and deepening
- relaxation and creation of a sense of well-being
- mind-over-body training
- ego-strengthening
- pain management via relaxation and transfer of warmth
- imagery training for healing
- post-hypnotic suggestions
- problem-solving skills
- self-hypnosis training.

Assessment and medical clearance

Before starting treatment it is important for the therapist to take a detailed clinical history and identify the essential psychological, physiological and social aspects of the patient's headache. This should include obtaining medical information and clearance from the patient's attending physician. It is crucial to rule out or identify organic etiology that may require medical intervention. However, it is recommended that the clinical assessment of the migraine patient be conducted within the context of the case formulation model.

As discussed in Chapter 2, the main function of a *case formulation* is to devise an effective treatment plan (*see* Appendices 2A and 2B). In order to identify the mechanisms that underlie the patient's migraine headache within the context of hypnotherapy, the eight-step case formulation (*see* Alladin, 2007) can be used. Table 4.1 summarizes the eight steps required to formulate the migraine case.

Education and establishment of rapport

The more understanding a patient has about his or her migraine and the treatment prescribed, the more collaborative the patient will be with the treatment, particularly as this sets the scene for the hypnotic induction. It is therefore vital to spend some time with the patient to provide the necessary information and answer any questions the patient may have. The TEAM approach described in Chapter 2 can be used to establish trust and rapport.

TABLE 4.1 Eight-step case formulation with migraine

1. List the major signs and symptoms of the migraine and indicate how they affect the functioning of the patient.
2. Formulate a formal diagnosis of the migraine and rule out organic causes.
3. Formulate a working hypothesis (e.g. whether the migraine is stress-related, due to over-arousal, or related to the patient's attitudes and beliefs).
4. Identify what triggers, exacerbates and maintains the migraine. Also identify the medication the patient may be on, noting the response to medication and the patient's 'pill-taking' behavior.
5. Explore the origin of the migraine and how it has affected the patient.
6. Summarize the working hypothesis.
7. Outline the treatment plan, integrating the pharmacological or other treatment the patient may be having.
8. Identify strengths and assets and predict obstacles to treatment.

Hypnotic induction and deepening

Any formal or informal method of hypnotic induction and deepening can be used. However, it is advisable to consider a few points before choosing an induction and deepening method. A patient with migraine may often have blurred vision or difficulty focusing, or may feel very anxious and irritable, and may be hypersensitive to various stimuli. A therapist should be aware of these factors and should therefore choose a hypnotic induction or deepening technique that does not require eye fixation or hyper-attentiveness, or any approach that is likely to further strain the patient. Also, if the initial hypnotic induction is recorded for making an audio cassette or CD to help the patient in self-hypnosis training, the induction technique needs to be simple and effective. I have adopted the relaxation with counting method from Gibbons (1979), which is easily adapted for self-hypnosis training (*see* Chapter 2, Appendix 2C for a complete script for induction and deepening).

Relaxation and creation of sense of well-being

As discussed above, the SAA model of migraine emphasizes the central role of sympathetic activity to account for most of the psychological, physiological and environmental factors known to be associated with migraine. According to the model, relaxation-related therapies and most anti-migraine drugs work by reducing sympathetic activity. One of the main objectives for using hypnosis is to induce a deep sense of relaxation. In terms of the SAA model, hypnosis reduces sympathetic arousal and induces parasympathetic dominance. By inducing relaxation, hypnosis reduces anxiety and thus makes it easier for patients to think about and discuss material they were previously too anxious to confront. Sometimes anxious and agitated patients are unable to pinpoint their maladaptive thoughts and emotions. However, once they close their eyes and relax, many of these same individuals appear to become more aware of their thoughts and feelings.

Through relaxation, hypnosis also reduces distraction and maximizes the patient's ability to concentrate, which can facilitate the learning of new material. Also, the induction of relaxation and 'creating a pleasant state of mind' (*see* Chapter 2, Appendix 2C) show migraine patients that they can relax, calm down and feel different. Such experience creates a sense of control and promotes positive expectancy of the treatment.

Mind-over-body training

The more credible and the more powerful the treatment is perceived to be by the patient, the better the treatment outcome (De Piano and Salzberg,1981). When the patient is in a fairly deep hypnotic trance, eye and body catalepsies (associated with the challenge to open eyes and get out of the chair or couch) are induced to demonstrate the power of the mind over the body. These demonstrations reduce scepticism over hypnosis and instil confidence in the migraine patients that they can produce significant emotional, behavioral and physiological changes.

This approach is exemplified by the case of Michael, a 40-year-old geologist with a 10-year history of chronic classic (with aura) migraine, who was referred to me for hypnotherapy by his neurologist. Michael was very sceptical of psychological treatment, especially hypnosis, for his migraine, which he considered to be a vascular disorder. The demonstration of the power of mind over body via eye and body catalepsies not only reduced his scepticism about hypnosis, but he also became a model patient and the frequency of his migraine attacks (from one per week to one attack every six weeks) significantly decreased after 12 sessions of hypnotherapy.

Ego-strengthening

Self-confidence and high self-esteem produce positive expectancy (Bandura, 1977). Ego-strengthening suggestions are offered to migraine patients to increase self-esteem and optimize treatment effect. The enhancement of feelings of self-esteem and self-efficacy can provide a powerful tool in working with migraine patients. Bandura (1977) has provided experimental evidence that *self-efficacy*, the expectation and confidence of being able to cope successfully with various situations, is one of the key elements in the effective treatment of phobic disorders. Individuals with a sense of high self-efficacy tend to perceive themselves as being in control. If migraine patients can be helped to view themselves as having the ability to control their symptoms, they will perceive the future as being hopeful.

The most popular method for increasing self-efficacy within the hypnotherapeutic context is to provide ego-strengthening suggestions. According to Hartland (1971), ego-strengthening suggestions 'remove tension, anxiety and apprehension, and . . . gradually restore the patient's confidence in himself and his ability to cope with his problems'. Hence his ego-strengthening suggestions (*see* Chapter 2, Appendix 2B) consist of generalized supportive suggestions to increase the patient's confidence, coping abilities, positive self-image and interpersonal skills.

However, to ensure credibility and acceptance of the ego-strengthening suggestions, it is of paramount importance that they be crafted in such a way that they appear credible and logical to the migraine patient. For example, rather than stating 'Your migraine will disappear', it is advisable to suggest something like the following.

EGO-STRENGTHENING IN MIGRAINE TREATMENT

As a result of this treatment and as a result of you listening to your self-hypnosis tape every day, you will begin to relax and learn to let go. And every day as you listen to your tape, you will begin to feel more and more deeply relaxed, less tense, less anxious, and less upset, so that every day your mind, your body, and your nerves will become more and more relaxed. As a result of this deep relaxation, every day, your mind, your body, and your nerves will become stronger and healthier. As a result of this, your migraines will become less frequent, less severe, until they will disappear completely.

This set of ego-strengthening suggestions not only sounds logical, but improvement becomes contingent on continuing with the therapy and listening to the self-hypnosis tape daily.

Pain management via relaxation and transfer of warmth

Hypnotherapy provides a powerful tool for producing a variety of cognitive, somatic, perceptual, physiological, visceral and kinesthetic changes under controlled conditions. Hypnotic production and modulation of these changes provide migraine patients with dramatic proof that they can change their feeling and experience, thus providing hope that they can alter their migraine symptoms. After two or three sessions of hypnosis and ego-strengthening, I begin to introduce relaxation and 'warming' techniques for symptom management.

RELAXATION FOR MIGRAINE SYMPTOM MANAGEMENT

You have now become so deeply relaxed and you are in such a deep trance, and your mind and your body feel so relaxed, so comfortable, that you can let yourself go completely. You begin to feel a sensation of peace and tranquility, relaxation and calm flowing all over your mind and body, giving you such a pleasant, and such a soothing sensation all over your mind and body, that you begin to feel all the tension, all the pressure easing away from your head. As you become more and more relaxed, you feel all the tension, all the pressure, all the discomfort easing away from your head. Soon you will feel so relaxed and so calm that your head will feel clear and comfortable.

The pain can be assessed and monitored through a 10-point scale (0 = no pain; 10 = worst pain) self-report. If a patient has a headache, it is useful to rate the pain before starting the hypnotherapy and then to monitor the level by regularly asking the rating from the patient. This monitoring of pain provides feedback both to the therapist and to the patient. If the pain goes during the session, the therapist can use the future tense when making suggestions of pain control. With chronic and severe migraine, relaxation suggestions may not be sufficient to ease the pain. Very often, the relaxation suggestions have to be integrated with the warming technique to create the desired effect.

RELAXATION AND WARMING FOR MIGRAINE SYMPTOM MANAGEMENT

You have now become so deeply relaxed, and you are in such a deep trance, and your mind has become so powerful, so sensitive to my suggestions, that you will be able to feel, imagine and experience everything I ask you to imagine, feel and experience. Now I want you to imagine yourself sitting in front of a bucket full of warm water. You know the water is warm because you can see the steam rising. (*It is advisable to monitor the patient's experience by regularly checking via an established ideomotor signal.*)

Become aware of the warm water surrounding your hand, dipped in the warm water. You feel the warmth from the water penetrating your hand and soon you will feel your hand feeling warm. When you feel your hand feel warm, let me know by nodding your head. (*I normally use the head-nod for YES and head shake for NO.*) As you focus on your hand, you begin to feel the warmth increasing, and soon you will feel a very warm feeling in your hand. You may begin to feel a tingling sensation in your hand. (*The therapist needs to wait until these changes occur; i.e. reported by the patient.*)

Now I want you to take your hand out of the warm water and gently rest your warm hand against your forehead. Gently massage your forehead, and as you do that you begin to feel the warmth from your hand spreading over your forehead. As you feel this warmth spreading over your forehead, you begin to feel your forehead becoming more and more relaxed, more and more comfortable. You will soon begin to feel the warmth spreading inside your head (*suggestions repeated until the patient can feel the warmth inside their head*).

As the warmth spreads inside your head, you feel your head becoming more and more relaxed, more and more comfortable, drifting into a deeper and deeper hypnotic trance. Soon you will feel so relaxed, so comfortable, that your head feels relaxed and comfortable, and as your head becomes more and more relaxed you feel all the tension, all the pressure, all the discomfort easing away from your head, and soon your head will feel clear and comfortable.

As a result of this hypnotic procedure, many migraine patients report dramatic reduction in their symptoms. De Piano and Salzberg (1981) believe such positive changes in patients are partly related to the rapid and profound behavioral, emotional, cognitive and physiological changes brought on by the induction of the hypnotic experience.

Imagery training for healing

Once the migraine patient is able to induce the warm feeling inside the head, the therapist capitalizes on this experience to promote healing and modification of the perceived underlying pathophysiology.

USING THE WARM FEELING TO PROMOTE HEALING

The warm feeling inside your head is due to the fact that the blood circulation inside your head has increased. Imagine the blood flow is increasing inside your head (*wait for the affirmative before proceeding further*). Imagine the extra blood flow is bringing in more oxygen and more nutrition to the areas where you need them. As a result of this extra blood, the tissues, the nerves, the arteries and the veins will become stronger and healthier, and as a result of this your migraines will become less frequent, less severe, until they will disappear completely.

Post-hypnotic suggestions

Post-hypnotic suggestions are provided to ratify the hypnotic experience, to promote self-hypnosis, and to counter problem behaviors, negative emotions and dysfunctional cognitions that may trigger or exacerbate the migraine symptoms. Post-hypnotic suggestions are a necessary part of the therapeutic process if the patient is to carry new possibilities into future experience (Yapko, 2003). Hence many clinicians use post-hypnotic suggestions to shape behavior.

Clarke and Jackson (1983) regard post-hypnotic suggestion as a form of 'higher-order conditioning', which functions as positive or negative reinforcement to increase or decrease the probability of desired or undesired behaviors, respectively. They have successfully utilized post-hypnotic suggestions to enhance the effect of *in vivo* exposure in agoraphobics. The following post-hypnotic suggestions can be used with migraine patients.

POST-HYPNOTIC SUGGESTIONS FOR MIGRAINE PATIENTS

As a result of this treatment, and as a result of you listening to your self-hypnosis tape every day, you will become less preoccupied with yourself, less preoccupied with your migraine, and less preoccupied with what you think other people think about you. As a result of this, every day you will become more and more interested in what you are doing and what is going on around you.

And every day as you listen to the tape, you will learn how to relax, how to let go, so that even when you have a headache, you will be able to relax. You will be able to unwind, relax and let go even when you have a headache. As a result of this, every day you will have more and more confidence controlling your headache, and you will become more and more confident coping with your migraine.

As a result of this treatment, you will also learn to warm your hand easily and quickly . . . so that when you have a headache you will be able to transfer the warmth to your head and the warmth will replace any discomfort you may have in your head. And also as you imagine the blood flow increasing inside your head, the nerves, the tissues and the blood vessels inside your head will become stronger and healthier. As a result of this your migraines will become less frequent, less severe, until they disappear completely.

Problem-solving skills

Migraine can be triggered, exacerbated and maintained by stress. The patients are therefore encouraged to identify physical (e.g. noise) and psychosocial (e.g. lack of assertiveness at work) problems or situations that can trigger, maintain or worsen the migraine symptoms. Various cognitive-behavioral techniques can be used to help migraine patients learn various strategies for coping with the triggering or maintaining factors. Hypnosis can be used to make the cognitive-behavioral strategies more experiential, and therefore more meaningful.

Self-hypnosis training

At the end of the first hypnotherapy session the patient is provided with an audio cassette or CD of self-hypnosis to practice at home. The homework assignment provides continuity of treatment between sessions and offers the patient the opportunity to learn self-hypnosis. The self-hypnosis component of the hypnotherapy is devised to induce relaxation, promote parasympathetic dominance, and provide tools for controlling the migraine symptoms. The self-hypnosis also helps to counter negative emotions, attitudes and behaviors.

Alman (2001) believes patients can achieve self-reliance and personal power by learning self-hypnosis. Yapko (2003) contends that teaching self-hypnosis and problem-solving strategies to patients allows them to develop self-correcting mechanisms that give them control over their lives.

COMPLEX CASES

Insight-oriented or exploratory hypnotic techniques can be used when the patient does not respond to the usual treatment protocol. This approach allows the therapist and the patient to explore intrapersonal dynamics and the unconscious origin or purposes of the migraine. There are many insight-oriented hypnotic methods (e.g. Brown and Fromm, 1986). The simplest and most widely used is ideomotor signaling. Hammond (1998, p. 114) introduces the ideomotor signaling to his hypnotized patient in the following manner.

IDEOMOTOR SIGNALING

We all have a conscious mind, and an unconscious mind; like a front of the mind, and a back of the mind. Your unconscious mind has tremendous capacity and power to help you. Your unconscious mind also knows a great deal about you, and sometimes it may be aware of things that we are not fully aware of consciously. And your unconscious mind can establish a method of signaling and communicating with us. Now I don't want you to consciously or voluntarily try to move or lift any of your fingers. But simply allow your unconscious mind, that it wishes to use as a signal for a response of 'yes.' And all by itself, entirely on its own, you'll simply discover one of those fingers developing a feeling of lightness, as if a helium balloon is attached with a string to the fingertip, and it will float up into the air all by itself. And just notice which finger begins to develop that light, floaty sensation, and then begins floating up, all by itself.

Your unconscious mind will select one of the fingers on your right/left hand that it wishes to use as a signal for 'yes.' And you'll notice a tendency to movement in one of those fingers. And you can just think over and over in your mind, 'yes, yes, yes,' and a finger will begin getting lighter, and lighter, and begin floating up.

Seven key areas can be explored with migraine patients using the ideomotor signaling technique:

❍ adaptive function or secondary gain for the symptoms

❍ self-punishment by having the migraine

❍ inner conflict causing the migraine

❍ imprints or commands transformed into migraine

❍ migraine as symbolic of past experiences

❍ migraine adopted as a form of identification

❍ migraine as symbolic of inner pain.

Once the underlying cause of the migraine is established, the therapist can help the patient deal with the issue in a satisfactory way. Migraine can also be compounded by comorbid psychiatric and/or medical problems. With these a comprehensive psychiatric and/or medical treatment will be required.

REFERENCES

Adams HE, Feuerstein M, Fowler JL. (1980). Migraine headache: review of parameters, etiology and intervention. *Psychological Bulletin* 87: 217–37.

Adelman JU, Adelman LC, Von Seggern R. (2002). Cost-effectiveness of antiepileptic drugs in migraine prophylaxis. *Headache* 42: 978–83.

Alladin A. (1991). *Psychological Factors in the Management of Migraine Headache.* Unpublished PhD dissertation, University of Manchester.

Alladin A. (2007). *Handbook of Cognitive Hypnotherapy for Depression: an evidence-based approach.* Philadelphia: Lippincott Williams and Wilkins.

Alman B. (2001). Self-care: approaches from self-hypnosis for utilizing your Unconscious (inner) potentials. In: Geary B, Zeig J, editors. *The Handbook of Ericksonian Psychotherapy* (pp. 522–40). Phoenix, AZ: The Milton H Erickson Foundation Press.

Anderson JAD, Basker MA, Dalton R. (1975). Migraine and hypnotherapy. *International Journal of Clinical and Experimental Hypnosis* 23(1): 48–58.

Andreychuk T, Skriver C. (1975). Hypnosis and biofeedback in the treatment of migraine headache. *International Journal of Clinical and Experimental Hypnosis* 23(3): 172–83.

Bakal DA. (1982). *The Psychology of Chronic Headache.* New York: Springer Publishing Company, Inc.

Bandura A. (1977). Self-efficacy: toward a unifying theory of behavioral change. *Psychological Review* 84 : 191–215.

Blanchard EB, Appelbaum KA, Guarnieri P, *et al.* (1997). Five year prospective follow-up on the treatment of chronic headache with biofeedback and/or relaxation. *Headache* 27: 580–3.

Brown D, Fromm E. (1986). *Hypnotherapy and Hypnoanalysis.* Hillside, NJ: Erlbaum.

Chambless D, Hollon SD. (1998). Defining empirically supported therapies. *Journal of Consulting and Clinical Psychology* 66: 7–18.

Cinciripini PM, Williamson DA, Epstein LH. (1981). Behavioral treatment of migraine headaches. In: Ferguson JM, Taylor CB, editors. *The Comprehensive Handbook of Behavioral Medicine* (vol. 2). New York: Spectrum Medical.

Clarke JC, Jackson JA. (1983). *Hypnosis and Behavior Therapy: the treatment of anxiety and phobias.* New York: Springer.

Dalessio DJ. (1980). *Wolff's Headache and Other Related Pain.* 4th ed. New York: Oxford University Press.

De Lozier JF, Gagnon RO. (1975). *National Ambulatory Medical Care Survey: 1973 summary: United States, May 1973–April 1974.* DHEW Publication No. HRA 76-1772. Washington DC: US Government Printing Office.

De Piano FA, Salzberg HC. (1981). Hypnosis as an aid to recall of meaningful information presented under three types of arousal. *International Journal of Clinical and Experimental Hypnosis* 29: 283–400.

Finer B. (1974). Clinical use of hypnosis in pain management. In: Bonica J, editor. *Advances in Neurology* (pp. 573–9). New York: Raven Press.

Feuerstein M, Gainer J. (1982). Chronic headache: etiology and management. In: Doleys DM, Meredith RL, Ciminero AR, editors. *Behavioral Medicine: assessment and treatment strategies*. New York: Plenum Press.

Gibbons DE. (1979). *Applied Hypnosis and Hyperempiria*. New York: Plenum Press.

Hammond DC. (1998). *Hypnotic Induction and Suggestion*. Chicago, Illinois: American Society of Clinical Hypnosis.

Hammond DC. (2007). Review of the efficacy of clinical hypnosis with headaches and migraines. *International Journal of Clinical and Experimental Hypnosis* 55: 207–19.

Hartland J. (1971). *Medical and Dental Hypnosis*. 2nd ed. London: Bailliere Tindall.

Headache Classification Committee of the International Headache Society. (2004). ICHD-II abbreviated pocket version. *Cephalalgia* 24(Suppl 1): 1–160.

Holroyd KA. (2002). Assessment and psychological management of recurrent headaches. *Journal of Consulting and Clinical Psychology* 70: 656–77.

Holyroyd KA, Andrasik F. (1982). A cognitive-behavioral approach to recurrent tension and migraine headache. In: Kendall PC, editor. *Advances in Cognitive-Behavioral Research and Therapy* (vol. 1). New York: Academic Press.

Mathew NT, Tfelt-Hansen P. (2006). General and pharmacologic approach to migraine management. In: Olesen J, Goadsby PJ, Ramadan NM, *et al.*, editors. *The Headaches*. 3rd ed (pp. 433–40). Philadelphia: Lippincott Williams and Wilkins.

Mathew RJ, Weinman ML, Largen JW. (1982). Sympathetic-adrenomedullary activation and migraine. *Headache* 22: 13–19.

McGrath PJ, Penzien D, Rains JC. (2006). Psychological and behavioral treatments of migraines. In: Olesen J, Goadsby PJ, Ramadan NM, *et al.*, editors. *The Headaches*. 3rd ed. (pp. 441–8). Philadelphia: Lippincott Williams and Wilkins.

Montgomery GH, Du Hamel KN, Redd WH. (2000). A meta-analysis of hypnotically induced analgesia: how effective is hypnosis? *International Journal of Clinical and Experimental Hypnosis* 48(2): 138–53.

National Institutes of Health. (1996). Technology Assessment Panel on Integration of Behavioral and Relaxation Approaches into the Treatment of Chronic Pain and Insomnia. *Journal of the American Medical Association* 276: 313–18.

Olesen J, Lipton BL. (2006). Classification of headache. In: Olesen J, Goadsby PJ, Ramadan NM, *et al.*, editors. *The Headaches*. 3rd ed. (pp. 9–15). Philadelphia: Lippincott Williams and Wilkins.

Philips C. (1978). Tension headache: theoretical problems. *Behavior Research and Therapy* 16: 249–61.

Spanos NP, Radtke-Bodorik HL, Ferguson JD, *et al.* (1979). The effects of hypnotic susceptibility, suggestions for analgesia and the utilization of cognitive strategies on the reduction of pain. *Journal of Abnormal Psychology* 88: 282–92.

Taylor FR, Martin VT. (2004). Migraine headache. In: Loder EW, Martin VT, editors. *Headache* (pp. 41–78). Philadelphia: American College of Physicians.

Yapko MD. (2003). *Trancework: an introduction to the practice of clinical hypnosis.* 3rd ed. New York: Brunner-Routledge.

Hypnotherapy with a Psychiatric Disorder: Depression

SUMMARY

This chapter describes the circular feedback model of depression (CFMD), which provides the rationale for combining hypnotherapy with cognitive-behavioral therapy (CBT) in the management of clinical depression. Cognitive hypnotherapy (CH), based on the model, provides a variety of treatment interventions for depression, from which a therapist can choose the best-fit strategies for a particular depressed client. CH also offers an innovative technique for developing antidepressive pathways. Although there is some empirical evidence for the effectiveness of CH, further studies are required before it can be established as an alternative treatment for depression.

INTRODUCTION

This chapter describes in detail how hypnotherapy can be integrated with cognitive behavior therapy (CBT) in the management of a severe emotional disorder – major depressive disorder (MDD). MDD is among one of the most common psychiatric disorders treated by psychiatrists and psychotherapists. Although MDD can be treated successfully with antidepressant medication and psychotherapy (Moore and Bona, 2001), a significant number of depressives do not respond to either medication or psychotherapy. It is therefore important for clinicians to continue to develop more effective treatments for depression.

Clinical depression also poses special problems to therapists because it is a complex disorder and it 'takes over the whole person – emotions, bodily functions, behaviors, and thoughts' (Nolen-Hoeksema, 2004, p. 280). This chapter will describe cognitive hypnotherapy (CH), a multimodal treatment approach to depression that may be applicable to a wide range of people with depression. The chapter also highlights the role of depressive rumination or negative self-hypnosis in the triggering, exacerbation and maintenance of the depressive disorder.

DESCRIPTION OF DEPRESSION

Depression is characterized by feelings of sadness, lack of interest in formerly enjoyable pursuits, sleep and appetite disturbance, feelings of worthlessness, and thoughts of death and dying (Alladin, 2007). Depression is extremely disabling in terms of poor quality of life and disability (Pincus and Pettit, 2001) and 15% of people with MDD commit suicide (Satcher, 2000). MDD is on the increase (World Health Organization, 1998), and it is estimated that out of every 100 people, approximately 13 men and 21 women are likely to develop the disorder at some point in their lives (Kessler *et al.*, 1994) and approximately one-third of the population may suffer from mild depression at some point in their lives (Paykel and Priest, 1992).

The prevalence rate of major depression is so high that the World Health Organization Global Burden of Disease Study ranked depression as the single most burdensome disease in the world in terms of total disability-adjusted life years among people in middle years of life (Murray and Lopez, 1996). According to the World Health Organization (1998), by the year 2020 clinical depression is likely to be second only to chronic heart disease as an international health burden, as measured by cause of death, disability, incapacity to work and medical resources used.

Major depression is a very costly disorder in terms of lost productivity at work, industrial accidents, bed occupancy in hospitals, treatment, state benefits and personal suffering. The illness also adversely affects interpersonal relationships with spouses and children (Gotlib and Hammen, 2002) and the rate of divorce is higher among depressives than among non-depressed individuals (e.g. Wade and Cairney, 2000). The children of depressed parents are at elevated risk of psychopathology (Gotlib and Goodman, 1999).

Approximately 60% of people who have a major depressive episode will have a second episode. Among those who have experienced two episodes, 70% will have a third, and among those who have had three episodes, 90% will have a fourth (American Psychiatric Association, 2000). Recurrence is very important in predicting the future course of the disorder as well as in choosing appropriate treatments. The median lifetime number of major depressive episodes is four, and 25% of depressives experience six or more episodes (Angst and Preizig, 1996). Depression is therefore considered to be a chronic condition that waxes and wanes over time but seldom disappears (Solomon *et al.*, 2000). The median duration of recurrent depression is five months.

Depression also co-occurs with other disorders, both medical and psychiatric. Kessler (2002), from his review of the epidemiology of depression, concludes that 'comorbidity is the norm among people with depression' (p. 29). For example, the Epidemiologic Catchment Area Study (Robins and Regier, 1991) found that 75% of respondents with lifetime depressive disorder also met criteria for at least one of the other DSM-III disorders assessed in that survey.

The most frequent comorbid condition with depression is anxiety, and in fact there is considerable symptom overlap between these two conditions. The presence of poor concentration, irritability, hypervigilance, fatigue, guilt, memory loss, sleep difficulties and worry may suggest a diagnosis of either disorder. The symptom overlap between the two conditions may indicate similar neurobiological correlates. At a psychological level it seems reasonable to assume that depression can result from the demoralization caused by anxiety; for example, in a case of an agoraphobic who becomes withdrawn because of the fear of going out. Conversely, a person with depression may become anxious due to worry about being unable to hold gainful employment.

Although there is an apparent overlap between anxiety and depression, it is common clinical practice to focus on treating one disorder at a time. The lack of an integrated approach to treatment means that a patient is treated only for depression while still suffering from anxiety. One of the rationales for combining hypnosis with cognitive behavior therapy, as described in this chapter, is to address symptoms of anxiety. The cognitive hypnotherapy approach to treatment described here is based on the author's experience of working with chronic depressives over the past 25 years.

TREATMENT OF DEPRESSION

In the past 20 years there have been significant developments and innovations in the pharmacological and psychological treatments of depression. The pharmacological, psychotherapeutic and hypnotherapeutic approaches to treatment are briefly reviewed below.

Pharmacotherapy

Over the past 20 years the tricyclics and the monoamine oxidase inhibitors (MAOIs) have been replaced by a second generation of antidepressants known as selective serotonin reuptake inhibitors (SSRIs), which have become extremely popular in the treatment of depression. Although these drugs are similar in structure to the tricyclics, they work more selectively to affect serotonin, which means the side-effects are less severe and they produce improvement within a couple of weeks. Moreover, these drugs are not fatal in overdose and they appear to help with a range of disorders, including anxiety, binge eating and premenstrual symptoms (Pearlstein *et al.*, 1997).

A number of other drugs such as Remeron, Serzone, Effexor and Wellbutrin have also been introduced during the past decade. They share some similarities with SSRIs, but they cannot be classified in any one of the previously mentioned categories. Sometimes these drugs are used in conjunction with SSRIs. Presently there is a variety of antidepressants available, but there are no consistent rules for determining which to use first. In clinical practice several antidepressants are often used before finding one drug that works well and with tolerable side-effects.

Antidepressant medications have relieved severe depression and undoubtedly prevented suicide in tens of thousands of patients around the world. Although these medications are readily available, many people refuse – or are not eligible – to take them. Some are wary of long-term side-effects. Women of childbearing age must protect themselves against the possibility of conceiving while taking antidepressants because they can damage the fetus. In addition, 40 to 50% of patients do not respond adequately to these drugs, and a substantial number of the remainder are left with residual symptoms of depression (Barlow and Durand, 2005, p. 238).

ECT is often given to patients who do not respond to drug therapies, and is known to relieve depression in 50 to 60% of depressives (Fink, 2001). ECT, however, remains a controversial treatment for several reasons, including cognitive and memory impairments, the idea of passing electrical current through a person's brain appears primitive, and it is still not known how ECT works.

Psychotherapy

Although antidepressant medications work well for many depressed patients, they obviously do not alleviate the problems that might have caused the depression in the first place. Bad marriages, unhappy work situations, or family conflicts that precede depression cannot be fixed by pills. Therefore, many depressed people benefit from psychotherapies designed to help them cope with the difficult life circumstances or personality vulnerabilities that put them at risk for depression. Psychotherapy is also indicated for people who have medical conditions (such as pregnancy and some heart problems) that preclude the use of medications.

Cognitive behavior therapy (CBT), which is the most popular psychosocial treatment for depression, has been studied in over 80 controlled trials (American Psychiatric Association, 2000). It has been found to be effective in the reduction of acute symptoms and compares favorably with pharmacological treatment among all but the most severely depressed patients. CBT also reduces relapse (Hollon and Shelton, 1991) and it can prevent the initial onset of the first episode or the emergence of symptoms in those at risk who have never been depressed (Gillham et al., 2000).

CBT is predicated on the notion that teaching patients to recognize and examine their negative beliefs and information-processing proclivities can produce relief from their symptoms and enable them to cope more effectively with life's challenges (Beck et al., 1979). The primary goal of the CBT therapist is to educate patients in the use of various techniques that allow them to examine their thoughts and modify maladaptive beliefs and behaviors. The main role of CBT is to help the patient learn to use these tools independently. Such skills are not only important for symptom relief, but may also minimize the chances of future recurrence of symptoms. The goals of CBT are achieved through a structured collaborative process consisting of three interrelated components: exploration, examination and experimentation (Hollon et al., 2002).

Hypnotherapy

Hypnosis has not been widely used in the management of clinical depression. The little published literature that exists can be categorized into case studies and adjunctive techniques. Alladin (2006, 2007) attributes the lack of progress in the application of hypnosis to depression to the myth created by some well-known writers that hypnosis can exacerbate suicidal behaviors in depressives. Alladin and Heap (1991) and Yapko (1992, 2001) have argued in response that hypnosis, especially when it forms part of a multimodal treatment approach, is not contraindicated with depression.

The bulk of the published literature on the clinical application of hypnosis to depression consists of case reports. These record the use of a variety of hypnotherapeutic techniques, but lack clarity on what therapists do with hypnosis in the management of depression (Burrows and Boughton, 2001). Nevertheless, several clinicians have used hypnosis as an adjunct to other forms of psychotherapy. For example, Golden *et al.* (1987), Tosi and Baisden (1984), Yapko (2001) and Zarren and Eimer (2001) have reported effective integration of CBT with hypnotherapy with depression in their clinical practice. However, with the exception of Alladin (1992a, 1992b, 1994; Alladin and Heap 1991), these writers have not provided a scientific rationale or a theoretical model for combining CBT with hypnosis in the management of clinical depression.

I have described a working model of non-endogenous depression which provides a theoretical framework for integrating cognitive and hypnotic techniques with depression (Figure 5.1). I revised the model (Alladin, 2007) and called it the circular feedback model of depression (CFMD). This model is briefly described below because it provides the theoretical underpinnings of the cognitive hypnotherapy for depression described in the rest of the chapter. The description of the model also highlights how hypnosis can be used as a useful construct to study and understand certain aspects of the depressive phenomenology.

COGNITIVE HYPNOTHERAPY FOR DEPRESSION

The CFMD gives three pragmatic reasons for combining cognitive and hypnotic paradigms in the treatment and understanding of depression. First, since hypnosis can produce cognitive, somatic, perceptual, physiological and kinesthetic changes under controlled conditions, the combination of the two paradigms may provide a conceptual framework for studying the psychological processes by which cognitive distortions produce concomitant psychobiological changes underlying clinical depression.

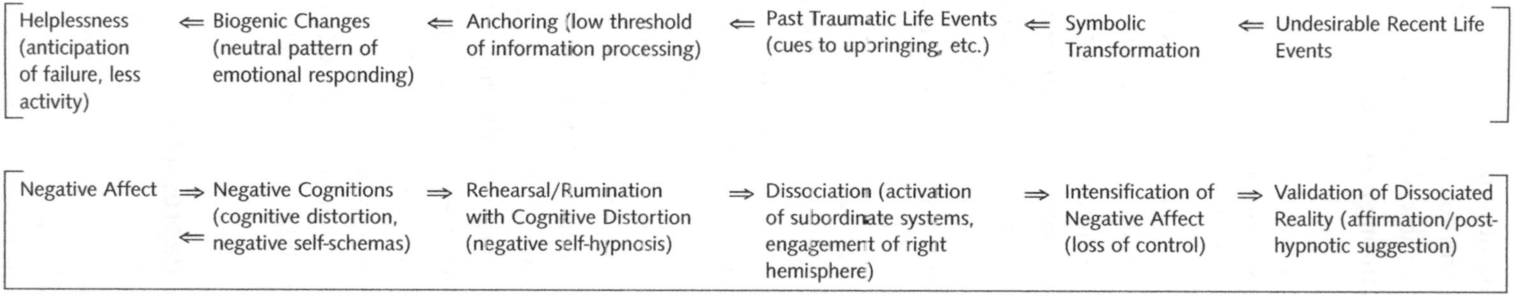

Helplessness (anticipation of failure, less activity) ⇐ Biogenic Changes (neutral pattern of emotional responding) ⇐ Anchoring (low threshold of information processing) ⇐ Past Traumatic Life Events (cues to upbringing, etc.) ⇐ Symbolic Transformation ⇐ Undesirable Recent Life Events

Negative Affect ⇒ Negative Cognitions (cognitive distortion, negative self-schemas) ⇐ Rehearsal/Rumination with Cognitive Distortion (negative self-hypnosis) ⇒ Dissociation (activation of subordinate systems, engagement of right hemisphere) ⇒ Intensification of Negative Affect (loss of control) ⇒ Validation of Dissociated Reality (affirmation/post-hypnotic suggestion)

Figure 5.1 Circular Feedback Model of Depression (CFMD) showing the constellation of 12 factors forming the depressive loop

Second, hypnosis provides insight into the phenomenology of depression (Yapko, 1992). Like hypnosis, depression is a highly subjective experience. It allows remarkable insights into the subjective realm of human experience, thus providing a paradigm for understanding how experience – normal or abnormal – is molded and patterned.

Third, after reviewing the strengths and limitations of CBT and hypnotherapy with depression, I concluded that each treatment approach has marked limitations (Alladin, 1989). For example, CBT does not allow access to unconscious cognitive restructuring, while hypnosis provides such access. On the other hand, hypnosis does not focus on systematic cognitive restructuring, while CBT's main focus is on cognitive restructuring via reasoning and Socratic dialogue. I have argued that some of the shortcomings of each treatment approach can be compensated for by integrating both treatment approaches (Alladin, 1989).

There is also some empirical evidence for combining hypnosis with CBT. Recently there has been a growing body of research evaluating the use of hypnosis with cognitive-behavioral techniques in the treatment of various psychological disorders. Schoenberger (2000), from her review of the empirical status of the use of hypnosis in conjunction with cognitive-behavioral treatment programmes, concluded that the existing studies demonstrate substantial benefits from the addition of hypnosis with cognitive-behavioral techniques. Similarly, Kirsch *et al.* (1995), from their meta-analysis of 18 studies comparing a cognitive-behavioral treatment with the same treatment supplemented by hypnosis, found the mean effect size of the difference between hypnotic and non-hypnotic treatment was 0.87 standard deviations. The authors concluded that hypnotherapy was significantly superior to non-hypnotic treatment.

I have just completed a study comparing the effects of CBT with cognitive hypnotherapy with 84 chronic depressives (Alladin and Alibhai, 2007). The results showed an additive effect of combining hypnosis with CBT. The study also met criteria for *probably efficacious* treatment for depression as laid down by the American Psychological Association Task Force (Chambless and Hollon, 1998), and it provides empirical validation for integrating hypnosis with CBT in the management of depression.

Circular feedback model of depression

The circular feedback model of depression (CFMD), which is a revised version of the cognitive dissociative model of depression (Alladin, 1994), was conceptualized to emphasize the bio-psychosocial nature of depression and to explicate the role of multiple factors that can trigger, exacerbate or maintain the depressive affect (Alladin, 2007). The model is not a new theory of depression or an attempt to explain the causes of depression. It is an extension of Beck's (1967) circular feedback model of depression, which was later elaborated by Schultz (1978, 1984, 2003) and Alladin (1994). In combining the cognitive and hypnotic paradigms, the CFMD incorporates ideas and concepts from information processing, selective attention, brain functioning, adverse life experiences, and the neodissociation theory of hypnosis (Hilgard, 1977).

The initial model was referred to as the cognitive dissociative model of depression because it encompassed the dissociative theory of hypnosis and proposed that non-endogenous depression was akin to a form of dissociation produced by negative cognitive rumination, which can be regarded as a form of negative self-hypnosis. The CFMD consists of 12 interrelated components that form a circular feedback loop (*see* Figure 5.1). The 12 components represent some of the major factors identified from the literature that may influence the course and outcome of depression. The components are described in detail elsewhere (*see* Alladin, 1994, 2006, 2007), so they are only briefly mentioned here to highlight the relationship among the 12 components forming the depressive loop.

The model attaches particular importance to the interaction between affect and cognition, and maintains there is a mutually reinforcing interaction between cognition and affect: thought influences feelings, but feelings too can influence thought content (hence the bi-directional arrows between negative affect and negative cognitions in Figure 5.1). The relationship between dysfunctional cognition and depressive affect is well documented in the literature (e.g. Haas and Fitzgibbon, 1989). An event (internal or external) can trigger a negative schema, which through cognitive rehearsal can lead to dissociation. In depression, Beck (1967, 1976) has noted patients' constant stereotypic preoccupation with their alleged negative personal attributes. I have argued (Alladin, 1992a) that such negative ruminations among some depressives is a form of negative self-hypnosis (Araoz 1981, 1985), which may lead to a state of partial or profound dissociation. Araoz (1981) regards negative self-hypnosis as the common denominator of all psychogenic problems.

Imagery is also considered by the model to be an important aspect of cognition in determining, maintaining and alleviating depression. Many writers (e.g. Ley and Freeman, 1984) claim that images have a greater capacity than language to attract and retrieve emotionally laden associations. Individuals predisposed to depression tend to focus on negative thoughts and images. Schultz (1978, 1984, 2003), Starker and Singer (1975) and Traynor (1974) have provided evidence that with increasing levels of depression, depressives tend to change the contents of their imagination to negative fantasies, and consequently are unable to redirect their thinking and imagery from their current problems and negative life concerns. In other words, the circular feedback cycle between cognition and affect repeats itself almost like a computer reverberating through an infinite loop (Schultz, 1978) as the depression worsens, thus validating the depressive reality in the form of self-affirmations or post-hypnotic suggestions. Neisser (1967) views such narrowing and distortion of the environment by a few repetitive behaviors and self-attributions as characteristic of psychopathology (i.e. there is an absence of reality testing).

The CFMD also attaches importance to both conscious and non-conscious information processing. Although we are capable of rational operations, most judgements are highly influenced by what is 'available' (particularly vivid information) in current memory at the time (Kahneman *et al.*, 1982). Shevrin and Dickman (1980), after reviewing the research evidence for non-conscious processes, concluded that no psychological model of human experience could ignore the concept of unconscious psychological processes. CBT, which relies on recognition and alteration of conscious cognition, may be ineffective here. Hypnosis provides a tool for accessing non-conscious information. Integration of non-conscious information processing within the CFMD widens our understanding, assessment and treatment of the depressive state. It was this realization that encouraged me to combine hypnosis with cognitive therapy. Several techniques for dealing with non-conscious cognitive influence are described under the treatment section.

Undesirable life events may further contribute to the maintenance of the depressive cycle (Schultz, 1978). However, Klinger (1975) points out that it is the 'symbolic transformation' of these events that is the critical factor. He suggests undesirable life events may serve as cues to past traumatic experiences. Depressives gradually not only become more sensitive to stimuli resembling past traumatic life events, but their reactions may also generalize to innocuous events or situations.

Such selective attending or 'anchoring' may explain the low threshold of information processing to emotional stimuli in depressives. Through repeated and automatic anchoring, biogenic changes may occur. Schwartz (1976, 1977, 1984) has provided evidence for the development of certain neurological pathways resulting from conscious cognitive focusing. It is feasible that depressives, through negative cognitive focusing, develop 'depressive pathways'. Individuals with anomalous developmental history (Guidano, 1987) and those who are biologically vulnerable (Oke *et al.*, 1978) or genetically predisposed to depression will be more prone to develop these depressive pathways.

When depressed, people with depression have the tendency to think more negatively (Beck *et al.*, 1979) and hence perceive the future as a continuous pattern of failure, relentless hardship and inability to cope. Such catastrophic preoccupation (negative self-hypnosis) promotes feelings of helplessness and hopelessness about the future. These feelings are further exacerbated if the individual lacks social skills (Youngren and Lewinshon, 1980), is surrounded by adverse environmental factors (Paykel *et al.*, 1969), or lacks social support (Brown and Harris, 1978). It is at this point in the depressive cycle that depressives are more vulnerable to suicide, or the depression can become more inflated, leading to aggravation of vegetative symptoms. Thus any of the 12 components in the loop can trigger depression, and the interrelationship among the factors allows the depressive loop to continue to reverberate. The purpose of therapy is to break the depressive loop and to learn a variety of skills to counter the factors that lead to the reverberation of the depressive cycle.

Treatment planning

The CFMD takes a multi-dimensional view of depression. The 12 factors forming the depressive loop are all interrelated, forming a constellation of emotional, cognitive, behavioral, physiological and non-conscious processes. Focusing on any of the factors allows the client and the therapist a point of entry into the depressive loop. Once the client and the therapist gain access into this set of relationships, they can deploy various techniques (some of these are described below) as tools to unravel and reorganize this interrelated set. Any of the factors can be used as a target for intervention, which can simultaneously influence other processes because of their interrelated nature (Simons *et al.*, 1984).

Because depression is a complicated disorder involving multiple factors, it is unlikely that a single causative factor – either biological or psychological – will be found. Therefore any single intervention is unlikely to be effective with every depressed patient. Although a clinical trial of CH has demonstrated that adding certain hypnotic techniques (hypnotic induction, relaxation, ego-strengthening, projection of problem-solving imagery and self-hypnosis) augments the effectiveness of CBT (Alladin and Alibhai, 2007), the treatment approach described below recommends multiple interventions. This is to encourage the therapist to develop a variety of techniques dealing with each factor, rather than being constrained by a few strategies.

This approach also reminds therapists that depression is often associated with various psychosocial difficulties and other comorbid conditions. Hence Williams (1992), in his comprehensive review of the psychotherapies for depression, concluded that the more techniques that are used, the more effective is the treatment. CH, based on the CFMD, provides a multi-factorial treatment approach to depression. A therapist can easily combine the most appropriate strategies to suit a particular patient.

STAGES OF COGNITIVE HYPNOTHERAPY

Cognitive hypnotherapy (CH) generally consists of 16 weekly sessions, which can be expanded or modified according to the patient's clinical needs, areas of concern and presenting symptoms. The stages of CH are described below. The sequence of the stages of treatment can be altered to suit the clinical needs of the individual patient.

Session 1: Clinical assessment

Before initiating CH it is important for the therapist to take a detailed clinical history to formulate the diagnosis and identify the essential psychological, physiological and social aspects of the patient's behaviors. The most efficient way to obtain all this information is to take a case formulation approach. The main function of a case formulation is to devise an effective treatment plan. The case formulation approach allows the clinician to translate and tailor a homothetic (general) treatment protocol to the individual (idiographic) patient.

I have described in great detail how to conduct cognitive hypnotherapy case formulation in order to select the most effective and efficient treatment strategies (Alladin, 2007). This approach emphasizes the role of cognitive distortions, negative self-instructions, irrational automatic thoughts and beliefs, schemas, and negative ruminations or negative self-hypnosis. By conceptualizing a case, the clinician develops a working hypothesis of how the patient's problems can be understood in terms of the cognitive-dissociative model. This understanding provides a compass or a guide to understanding the treatment process. The evidence suggests that matching treatment to particular patient characteristics improves outcome (Beutler *et al.*, 2000).

Session 2: First aid for depression

Depressives tend to be plagued by feelings of low mood, hopelessness and pessimism, so any immediate relief from these feelings provides a sense of hope and optimism. Alladin (1994, 2006, 2007) and Overlade (1986) have described a first aid technique for producing immediate relief from the pervasive depressed feeling. The goal of first aid is to:

❍ break the depressive cycle

❍ produce positive (non-depressive) feelings

❍ develop anti-depressive pathways

❍ establish therapeutic alliance

❍ produce positive expectancy in the client.

The first aid technique consists of seven stages (*see* Alladin, 2006, 2007 for a detailed description). This technique is particularly effective with a patient who becomes acutely depressed in response to situational stressors such as injustice or being treated unfairly by a spouse. The first aid serves as a crisis intervention, but is specifically devised to alter depressive affect. The first aid for depression can be used with or without hypnotic induction. Following are the seven stages:

1. The patient is encouraged to talk about the situational factor that triggered or exacerbated the depressive affect and is then allowed to ventilate feelings of distress and frustration.
2. A plausible biological explanation (a 'tucking reflex') of acute depression is provided to reduce guilt for feeling depressed.
3. The patient is helped to alter the depressive posture or 'tucking response' by holding the head high and squaring the shoulders (advised to adopt the posture of a soldier on guard).
4. The patient is encouraged to make deliberate attempts to smile by imagining looking in a mirror.
5. The patient is encouraged to imagine a 'funny face'.
6. The patient is encouraged to 'play a happy mental tape'.
7. The patient is conditioned to a positive cue word (e.g. 'bubbles') that will conjure a smile.

Sessions 3 to 6: Cognitive behavior therapy (CBT)

At least four sessions are devoted to cognitive behavior therapy (CBT). The object of the CBT sessions is to help the patients identify and restructure their dysfunctional beliefs that may be triggering and maintaining their depressive affect. CBT techniques are fully described in several excellent books (e.g. Beck, 1995) so they are not described in detail here. Within the CH framework I have found the following sequential presentation of the CBT components to be beneficial to depressed patients (Alladin, 2006).

○ The patient is offered a practical explanation of the cognitive model of depression.

○ The patient is advised to read the first three chapters from *Feeling Good: the new mood therapy* (Burns, 1999).

○ The patient is encouraged to identify the cognitive distortions that form part of their negative rumination.

○ The patient is advised to record their thoughts and feelings on the ABC form (a form with three columns: A = event; B = automatic thoughts; C = emotional responses). This homework helps the patient discover the link between thoughts and feelings.

○ The patient is introduced to the concept of disputation (D) or challenging of cognitive distortions after they have had the opportunity to log the ABC form for a week.

○ The ABCDE form is introduced to log disputation and the effects of disputation over negative affect. This form is an expanded version of the ABC form, by including two more columns (D = disputation; E = consequences of disputation).

○ The patient is provided with a completed version (with disputation of cognitive distortions in column D and the modification of emotional and behavioral responses in column E as a consequence of cognitive disputation) of the ABCDE form as an example of disputation.

○ The patient is coached to differentiate between superficial ('I can't do this') and deeper ('I'm a failure') dysfunctional beliefs (negative self-schemas).

○ The patient is coached on how to access and restructure deeper self-schemas.

○ The patient is advised to constantly monitor and restructure negative cognition until it becomes a habit.

The number of CBT sessions is determined by the needs of the patient and the presentation of symptoms. The CBT sessions prepare the patient for cognitive restructuring under hypnosis (*see* sessions 9 to 12).

Sessions 7 to 8: Hypnosis

Formal hypnosis is introduced in sessions 7 and 8, although a brief induction procedure may be used to facilitate the first aid technique in the second session. I have argued for the following reasons for utilizing hypnosis within the CH framework (Alladin, 2006); hypnosis:

○ induces relaxation

○ reduces distraction

○ maximizes concentration

○ facilitates divergent thinking

○ amplifies experiences

○ provides access to non-conscious psychological processes.

The focus of the first two hypnotic sessions is on (a) relaxation (to prove to the patient that he or she can relax), (b) somatosensory changes (to reinforce the idea that the patient can have different feelings and sensations), (c) demonstration of the power of the mind (via eye and body catalepsy), (d) ego-strengthening, and (e) increasing confidence in the ability to utilize self-hypnosis.

Ego-strengthening is a very important component of the hypnotic sessions. Ego-strengthening is 'a way of exploiting the positive experience of hypnosis and the therapist–patient relationship to develop feelings of confidence and optimism and an improved self-image' (Alladin and Heap, 1991, p. 58). When a satisfactory deep level of 'trance' is achieved, a modified version of Hartland's (1971) ego-strengthening suggestions is given. To ensure acceptance of these suggestions, it is of paramount importance to first create a positive mental set and a 'pleasant state of mind'. Moreover, the ego-strengthening suggestions need to be plausible and logical.

For instance, rather than stating 'Every day you will feel better', it is better to suggest, 'As a result of this treatment and as a result of you listening to your self-hypnosis tape every day, you will begin to feel better'. This set of suggestions not only sounds logical, but improvement becomes contingent on continuing with the therapy and listening to the self-hypnosis tape daily. Here are some examples of the ego-strengthening suggestions adapted from Alladin, 2006 (pp. 161–2).

SUGGESTIONS FOR EGO-STRENGTHENING

- Day by day, as you listen to your self-hypnosis tape, you will become more relaxed, less anxious, and less depressed.
- As a result of this treatment and as a result of you listening to your self-hypnosis tape every day, you will begin to feel more confident and you will begin to cope better with the changes and challenges of life every day.
- You will begin to focus more and more on your achievements and successes than on your failures and shortcomings.

Patients are also offered post-hypnotic suggestions just before the end of the hypnosis session to counter negative self-hypnosis (NSH). Depressives tend to constantly ruminate on negative thoughts, feelings and images (a form of NSH), especially after a negative affective experience (e.g. 'I will not be able to cope'). This can be regarded as a form of negative post-hypnotic suggestion, which can become part of the depressive cycle. To break the depressive cycle it is very important to counter the NSH. Here are some examples of post-hypnotic suggestion for countering NSH (Alladin, 2006, p. 162).

EXAMPLES OF POST-HYPNOTIC SUGGESTION FOR COUNTERING NEGATIVE SELF-HYPNOSIS

- While you are in an upsetting situation, you will become more aware of how to deal with it rather than focusing on your depressed feeling.
- When you plan and take action to improve your future, you will feel more optimistic about the future.
- As you feel involved in doing things, you will be motivated to do more things.

At the end of the first hypnosis session the patient is provided with an audiotape of self-hypnotic procedures for inducing relaxation and creating a positive mental set and a good frame of mind. The self-hypnosis tape also consists of ego-strengthening suggestions and post-hypnotic suggestions. The homework assignment provides continuity of treatment between sessions and offers the patient the opportunity to learn self-hypnosis.

Sessions 9 to 12: Cognitive reframing under hypnosis

The next three sessions integrate the CBT and hypnotic strategies learned so far, and also address non-conscious schemas. More specifically, the sessions focus on cognitive restructuring under hypnosis, expansion of awareness and amplification of experiences, and reduction of guilt and self-blame.

Cognitive restructuring under hypnosis

Hypnosis provides a powerful vehicle for exploring and expanding cognitive distortions below the level of awareness. Sometimes in the course of CBT the patient reports being unable to access cognitions preceding depressive affect. Hypnosis provides access to unconscious cognitive distortions and negative self-schemas, so unconscious maladaptive cognitions can be easily retrieved and restructured under hypnosis. This is achieved by directing the patient's attention to the psychological content of an experience or situation.

The patient is guided to focus attention on a specific area of concern and to establish the link between cognition and affect. Once the negative cognitions are identified, the patient is encouraged to restructure the maladaptive cognitions and then attend to the resulting (desirable) responses. For instance, if a person reports, 'I don't know why I felt depressed at the party last week', the patient is hypnotically regressed back to the party and encouraged to identify and restructure the faulty cognitions until the patient can think of the party without being upset.

I used this procedure effectively to treat a depressed patient, Rita, who was unable to identify the cognitions related to social and sexual withdrawal, which were interfering with her relationship with her husband (Alladin, 2006). The following transcript (pp. 164–5) describes the hypnotic procedure of accessing and restructuring non-conscious cognitive schemas.

> *Therapist: I would like you to go back in time and place in your mind to last Tuesday night when you felt upset and wanted to withdraw yourself from your husband. (Pause) Take your time. Once you are able to remember the situation, let me know by nodding your chin up and down. (ideomotor signals of 'chin up and down for YES' and 'shaking your head side to side for NO' were set up prior to starting the regression).*

After a short while, she nodded her chin.

> *Become aware of the feelings, allowing all the feelings to flow through you. Become aware of your bodily reactions. Become aware of every emotion you feel.*

Her breathing and heart rate increased and the muscles in her face started to contract. It became noticeable that she was feeling upset and anxious.

How do you feel? (Pause) Take your time, and you can speak up; speaking will not disturb your trance level.

Rita: I'm scared . . . it's unfair . . . no one told me he was going to be sent away. (She started to cry.)

Rita recounted two traumatic incidents that occurred when she was 10 and 12 years old respectively. When she was 10 years old, her brother Ken (two years older than her) was sent away to live with her grandparents. Ken was supposedly a very naughty child and the parents could not handle him so they 'got rid of him'. Rita was very distressed by it because she was very close to Ken and 'they never told her that Ken was going to be sent away'. She cried for days and for several nights she could not sleep. One night while she was lying in her bed at night, the thought of a dark cave came into her mind and she saw herself being in that dark cave. Although it was frightening initially, later on she felt a sense of comfort, she felt closed in and she did not have to think of anything or feel anything. From this night, whenever she felt upset she would go into the cave in her mind and lock herself in. The second incident happened two years later. One Saturday morning the family got the news that Ken (who was still living with grandparents) died from drowning in the local swimming pool. Immediately, it flashed in her mind that she lost the person she loved most. She felt very upset, but only briefly, because she quickly locked herself in the 'dark cave'. From the regression it became apparent that (a) Rita retreats to the dark cave whenever she feels confronted or stressed out, and (b) she is fearful of getting closer to anyone who loves her (including her husband) in case she loses that person.

Therapist: I want you to come back to Tuesday night when you felt upset. I want you to become aware of the thoughts and images that were going in your mind.

Rita: I can't deal with this. It's too painful. I'll lose him. I don't want to lose him. (She started to cry.)

Therapist: From now on you will become completely aware of all the thoughts that go in your mind when you are upset so that you begin to see the connection between your thinking and your feeling.

The procedure helped Rita to identify the unconscious negative cognitions associated with her upsetting feeling and, consequently, she was able to restructure her thinking and control her emotional and behavioral reactions.

Two further sessions were used to help Rita deal with the two uncovered traumatic events. Her negative experience and the associated faulty cognitions were 'reframed' by utilizing her adult ego state (she was able to reflect on the incidents utilizing her 'adult ego lenses'). Following these sessions Rita's anxiety and sexual difficulties dramatically improved. Through her 'adult ego lenses' she was able conceptualize that it was no longer necessary for her to retreat into the dark cave and she realized there is no direct relationship between loving and losing. Consequently, her relationship with her husband significantly improved. Other hypnotic uncovering or restructuring procedures such as affect bridge, age regression, age progression and dream induction can also be used to explore and restructure negative schemas.

Expansion of awareness and amplification of experiences

Hypnosis provides a powerful device for expanding awareness and amplifying experience. Brown and Fromm (in Hammond, 1990, pp. 322–4) describe a technique called 'enhancing affective experience and its expression' for expanding and intensifying positive feelings. The object of this procedure is to help depressed patients create, amplify and express a variety of negative and positive feelings and experience. Enhancing affective experience and its expression is specifically devised to (a) bring underlying emotions into awareness, (b) create awareness of various feelings, (c) intensify positive affect, (d) enhance 'discovered' affect, (e) induce positive moods, and (f) increase motivation. Such a technique not only disrupts the depressive cycle but also helps to develop antidepressive pathways.

An underlying emotion can be brought into awareness by suggesting to the hypnotized patient: 'When I count from ONE to FIVE . . . by the time you hear me say FIVE . . . you will begin to feel whatever emotion is associated with your depressive feeling.' Then the patient is encouraged to amplify the affect by stating, 'When I count slowly from ONE to FIVE . . . as I count you will begin to feel that feeling more and more intensely . . . so that when I reach the count of FIVE . . . at the count of FIVE you will feel it in your body as strongly as you can bear it . . . Now notice what you feel and you will be able to describe it to me.'

The procedure can be easily extended by regressing the patient to past and future projections.

Reduction of guilt and self-blame

In some patients, depression is often maintained by 'old garbage' such as guilt and self-regrets. Various hypnotherapeutic techniques can be utilized to reframe the patient's past experience that causes guilt or self-regrets. Hammond (1990) provides several techniques for dealing with guilt and self-blame. For example, Watkins (in Hammond, 1990, p. 312) describes a technique she calls 'the door of forgiveness' for reducing guilt, and Hammond and Stanton (in Hammond, 1990, p. 313) describe two techniques for 'dumping the rubbish'. One of Stanton's dumping-the-rubbish techniques is 'the laundry' technique.

The laundry technique involves, when in deep trance, imagining (a) a laundry, (b) filling the sink with water, (c) opening a trap door in the head, (d) pulling out the unwanted rubbish (guilt, self-blame and self-regrets) from the brain and dumping it into the water, (e) the water turning blacker and blacker, and (f) finally, pulling the plug, allowing the dirty water (guilt, self-blame and self-regrets) to drain away. Although simple, this metaphor works very well.

Session 9: Attention switching and positive mood induction

Depressives have the tendency to become preoccupied with catastrophic thoughts and images. Such ruminations can easily become obsessional and may also kindle the brain to develop depressive pathways, thus impeding therapeutic progress. To counter the development of depressive pathways the positive mood induction technique is used and attention-switching exercises are devised to break the negative ruminative cycle. These techniques are briefly described below.

Developing antidepressive pathways

Just as the brain can be kindled to produce depressive pathways through conscious negative focusing (Schwartz *et al.*, 1976), the brain can also be kindled to develop antidepressive or happy pathways by focusing on positive imagery (Schwartz, 1984). There is extensive empirical evidence that directed cognition can produce neuronal changes in the brain and that positive affect can enhance adaptive behavior and cognitive flexibility (*see* Alladin, 2007). Within this theoretical and empirical context, I have devised the positive mood induction technique to counter depressive pathways and to develop antidepressive pathways (Alladin 1994, 2006, 2007). Apart from providing a systematic approach for developing antidepressive pathways, the technique also fortifies the brain to withstand depressive symptoms, thus preventing relapse and recurrence of future depressive episodes.

The positive mood induction technique consists of four steps: (1) education, (2) making a list of positive experiences, (3) positive mood induction, (4) post-hypnotic suggestions, and (5) home practice. To educate the patient, the therapist provides a scientific rationale for producing antidepressive pathways. The patient is then advised to make a list of 10 to 15 pleasant or positive experiences. When in deep trance, the patient is instructed to focus on a positive experience from the list of positive experiences, which is then amplified with assistance from the therapist. The technique is very similar to enhancing affective experience and its expression. However, to develop antidepressive pathways, more emphasis is placed on producing somatosensory changes in order to induce more pervasive concomitant physiological changes. The procedure is repeated with at least three positive experiences from the list of pleasant experiences. Post-hypnotic suggestions are provided so that the patient, with practice, will be able to regress completely when practicing at home with the list.

Attention switching

The patient is encouraged to practice with the list four to five times a day. In addition, the patient is encouraged to switch off from negative rumination as soon as he or she becomes aware of it, and to replace it by one of the items from his or her 'pleasant' list. This procedure provides another technique for weakening the depressive pathways and strengthening the 'happy pathways'. In other words, the patient learns to substitute negative self-hypnosis with positive self-hypnosis. Yapko (1992) argues that since depressives utilize negative self-hypnosis to create the experience of the depressive reality, they can equally learn to use positive self-hypnosis to create an experience of antidepressive reality.

Session 13: Active interactive training

This technique helps to break 'dissociative' habits and encourages 'association' with the relevant environment. When interacting with their internal or external environment, depressives tend to passively dissociate rather than actively interact with the relevant external information. Active interaction means being alert and 'in tune' with the incoming information (conceptual reality), whereas passive dissociation is the tendency to anchor to 'inner reality' (negative schemas and associated syncretic feelings), which inhibits reality testing or appraisal of conceptual reality.

To prevent passive dissociation, a person must (1) become aware of such a process occurring, (2) actively attempt to inhibit it by switching attention away from 'bad anchors', and (3) actively attend to relevant cues or conceptual reality.

In other words, the patient learns to actively engage the dominant hemisphere by becoming analytical, logical, realistic and syntactical. Edgette and Edgette (1995, pp. 145–58) have also discussed several techniques for developing adaptive dissociation. For example, a patient with habitual maladaptive dissociation can be trained to embrace adaptive dissociation, which helps to counter maladaptive dissociation, halt a sense of pessimism and sense of helplessness, and detach from toxic self-talk.

Session 14: Social skills training

Youngren and Lewinshon (1980) have provided evidence that lack of social skills may cause and maintain depression in some patients. A session (or more sessions if required) is therefore devoted to teaching social skills, and the patient is advised to read the appropriate bibliography. The social skills training can be enhanced by hypnosis via imagery training and imaginal rehearsal.

Session 15 to 16: Ideal goals/reality training

Under hypnosis the patient is encouraged to image ideal but realistic goals, and then to imagine planting appropriate strategies and taking necessary actions for achieving them (forward projection with behavioral rehearsal).

Booster and follow-up sessions

Cognitive therapy, as outlined above, normally requires 16 weekly sessions. Some clients may, however, require fewer or more sessions. After these sessions, further booster or follow-up sessions may be provided as required.

REFERENCES

Abramson LY, Alloy LB, Hankin BL, *et al.* (2002). Cognitive-vulnerability: stress models of depression in a self-regulatory and psychobiological context. In: Gotlib IH, Hammen CL, editors. *Handbook of Depression* (pp. 268–94). New York: Guilford Press.

Alladin A. (1989). Cognitive-hypnotherapy for depression. In: Waxman D, Pederson D, Wilkie I, *et al.*, editors. *Hypnosis: the 4th European Congress at Oxford* (pp. 175–82). London: Whurr Publishers.

Alladin A. (1992a). Depression as a dissociative state. *Hypnos: Swedish Journal of Hypnosis in Psychotherapy and Psychosomatic Medicine* 19: 243–53.

Alladin A. (1992b). Hypnosis with depression. *American Journal of Preventive Psychiatry and Neurology* 3(3): 13–18.

Alladin A. (1994). Cognitive hypnotherapy with depression. *Journal of Cognitive Psychotherapy: An International Quarterly* 8(4): 275–88.

Alladin A. (2007). *Handbook of Cognitive Hypnotherapy for Depression: an evidence-based approach.* Philadelphia: Lippincott Williams and Wilkins.

Alladin A, Alibhai A. (2007). Cognitive-hypnotherapy for depression: an empirical investigation. *International Journal of Clinical and Experimental Hypnosis*, 55: 147–66.

Alladin A, Heap M. (1991). Hypnosis and depression. In: Heap M, Dryden W, editors. *Hypnotherapy: a handbook* (pp. 49–67). Milton Keynes: Open University Press.

American Psychiatric Association. (1980). *Diagnostic and Statistical Manual of Mental Disorders.* 3rd ed. Washington, DC: American Psychiatric Association.

American Psychiatric Association. (1994). *Diagnostic and Statistical Manual of Mental Disorders.* 4th ed. Washington, DC: American Psychiatric Association.

American Psychiatric Association. (2000). *Diagnostic and Statistical Manual of Mental Disorders.* 4th ed., text rev. Washington, DC: American Psychiatric Association.

Angst J, Preizig M. (1996). Course of a clinical cohort of unipolar, bipolar and schizoaffective patients: results of a prospective study from 1959 to 1985. *Schweizer Archiv fur Neurologie und Psychiatrie* 146: 1–16.

Araoz DL. (1981). Negative self-hypnosis. *Journal of Contemporary Psychotherapy* 12: 45–52.

Araoz DL. (1985). *The New Hypnosis.* New York: Brunner/Mazel Publishers.

Barber TX, Wilson SC. (1978–79). The Barber suggestibility scale and the creative imagination scale: experimental and clinical applications. *American Journal of Clinical Hypnosis* 21: 85.

Barlow DH, Durand VM. (2005). *Abnormal Psychology: an integrative approach.* 4th ed. London: Thomson Wadsworth.

Beck AT. (1967). *Depression: clinical, experimental and theoretical aspects*. New York: Hoeber.

Beck AT. (1976). *Cognitive Therapy and Emotional Disorders*. New York: International University Press.

Beck AT, Rush AJ, Shaw BF, *et al.* (1979). *Cognitive Therapy of Depression*. New York: Guilford Press.

Beck AT, Steer RA. (1993a). *Beck Anxiety Inventory*. San Antonio, TX: Harcourt Brace.

Beck AT, Steer RA. (1993b). *Beck Hopelessness Scale*. San Antonio, TX: Harcourt Brace.

Beck AT, Steer RA, Brown KB. (1996). *The Beck Depression Inventory – Revised*. San Antonio, TX: Harcourt Brace.

Beck AT, Young JE. (1985). Depression. In: Barlow DH, editor. *Clinical Handbook of Psychological Disorders*. New York: Guilford Press.

Beck J. (1995). *Cognitive Therapy: basics and beyond*. New York: Guilford Press.

Beutler LE, Clarkin JE, Bongar B. (2000). *Guidelines for the Systematic Treatment of the Depressed Patient*. New York: Oxford University Press.

Bower G. (1981). Mood and memory. *American Psychologist* 36: 129–48.

Brown DP, Fromm E. (1990). Enhancing affective experience and its expression. In: Hammond DC, editor. *Hypnotic Suggestions and Metaphors* (pp. 322–4). New York: WW Norton and Company.

Brown GW, Harris, T. (1978). *Social Origins of Depression*. New York: Free Press.

Burns DD. (1999). *Feeling Good: the new mood therapy*. New York: Avon Books.

Burrows GD, Boughton SG. (2001). Hypnosis and depression. In: Burrows GD, Stanley RO, Bloom PB, editors. *International Handbook of Clinical Hypnosis* (pp. 129–42). New York: John Wiley and Sons, Ltd.

Chambless DL, Hollon SD. (1998). Defining empirically supported therapies. *Journal of Consulting and Clinical Psychology* 66: 7–18.

Coryell W, Leon A, Winokur G, *et al.* (1996). Importance of psychotic features to long-term course in major depressive disorder. *American Journal of Psychiatry* 153: 483–9.

Dobson KS. (1986). The self-schema in depression. In: Hartmen LM, Blankstein KR, editors. *Perception of Self in Emotional Disorder and Psychotherapy* (pp. 187–217). New York: Plenum Press.

Edgette JH, Edgette JS. (1995). *The Handbook of Hypnotic Phenomena in Psychotherapy*. New York: Brunner/Mazel Publishers.

Fava M, Rosenbaum JF. (1995). Pharmacotherapy and somatic therapies. In: Beckham EE, Leber WR, editors. *Handbook of Depression*. 2nd ed. (pp. 280–301). New York: Guilford Press.

Fink M. (2001). Convulsive therapy: a review of the first 55 years. *Journal of Affective Disorders* 63: 1–15.

Gibbons DE. (1979). *Applied Hypnosis and Hyperempiria*. New York: Plenum Press.

Gillham JE, Shatte AJ, Freres DR. (2000). Preventing depression: a review of cognitive-behavioral and family interventions. *Applied and Preventive Psychology* 9: 63–88.

Golden WL, Dowd ET, Friedberg F. (1987). *Hypnotherapy: a modern approach*. New York: Pergamon Press.

Gotlib IH, Goodman SH. (1999). Children of parents with depression. In: Silverman WK, Ollendick TH, editors. *Developmental Issues in the Clinical Treatment of Children* (pp. 415–32). Boston: Allyn and Bacon.

Gotlib IH, Hammen CL. (2002). Introduction. In: Gotlib IH, Hammen CL, editors. *Handbook of Depression* (pp. 1–20). New York: Guilford Press.

Guidano VF. (1987). *Complexity of the Self: a developmental approach to psychopathology and therapy*. New York: Guilford Press.

Haas GL, Fitzgibbon ML. (1989). In: Mann JJ, editor. *Models of Depressive Disorders* (pp. 9–43). New York: Plenum Press.

Hamilton M. (1967). Development of a rating scale for primary depressive illness. *British Journal of Social and Clinical Psychology* 6: 278–96.

Hammond DC, editor. (1990). *Handbook of Hypnotic Suggestions and Metaphors*. New York: WW Norton and Company.

Hartland J. (1971). *Medical and Dental Hypnosis and its Clinical Applications*. 2nd ed. London: Bailliere Tindall.

Hilgard ER. (1977). *Divided Consciousness: multiple controls in human thought and action*. New York: John Wiley and Sons.

Hollon SD, Haman KL, Brown LL. (2002). Cognitive-behavioral treatment of depression. In: Gotlib IH, Hammen CC, editors. *Handbook of Depression* (pp. 383–403). New York: Guilford Press.

Hollon SD, Shelton M. (1991). Contributions of cognitive psychology to assessment and treatment of depression. In: Martin PR, editor. *Handbook of Behavior Therapy and Psychological Science: an integrated approach* (vol. 164, pp. 169–95). New York: Pergamon Press.

Horowitz MJ. (1972). Image formation: clinical observation and a cognitive model. In: Sheehan PW, editor. *The Function and Nature of Imagery* (pp. 282–309). New York: Academic Press.

Janet P. (1889). *L'Automatisme Psychologique*. Paris: Felix Alcan.

Janet P. (1907). *The Major Symptoms of Hysteria*. New York: Macmillan.

Jaynes J. (1976). *The Origin of Consciousness in the Breakdown of the Bicameral Mind*. Boston: Houghton Mifflin Co.

Kahneman D, Slovic P, Tversky A. (1882). *Judgment Under Uncertainty: heuristics and biases*. Cambridge: Cambridge University Press.

Kessler RC. (2002). Epidemiology of depression. In: Gotlib IH, Hammen CC, editors. *Handbook of Depression* (pp. 23–42). New York: Guilford Press.

Kessler RC, McGongale KA, Zhao S, *et al.* (1994). Lifetime and 12-month prevalence of DSM-III-R psychiatric disorders in the United States: results from the National Comorbidity Survey. *Archives of General Psychiatry* 51: 8–19.

Kirsch I, Montgomery G, Sapirstein G. (1995). Hypnosis as an adjunct to cognitive-behavioral psychotherapy: a meta-analysis. *Journal of Consulting and Clinical Psychology* 63: 214–20.

Klinger E. (1975). The nature of fantasy and its clinical uses. In: Klinger JL, Chair. *Imagery Approaches to Psychotherapy*. Symposium presented at the Meeting of the American Psychological Association, Chicago.

Ley RG, Freeman RJ. (1984). Imagery, cerebral laterality, and the healing process. In: Sheikh AA, editor. *Imagination and Healing* (pp. 51–68). New York: Baywood Publishing Co. Inc.

Moore JD, Bona JR. (2001). Depression and dysthymia. *Medical Clinics of North America* 85(3): 631–44.

Murray CJL, Lopez AD, editors. (1996). *The Global Burden of Disease: a comprehensive assessment of mortality and disability from diseases, injuries, and risk factors in 1990 and projected to 2020*. Cambridge, MA: Harvard University Press.

Neisser U. (1967). *Cognitive Psychology*. New York: Appleton-Century-Croft.

Nemeroff CB. (2000). An ever-increasing pharmacopoeia for the management of patients with bipolar disorder. *Journal of Clinical Psychiatry* 61(Suppl. 13): 19–25.

Nolen-Hoeksema S. (2004). *Abnormal Psychology*. 3rd ed. New York: The McGraw-Hill Companies.

Oke A, Keller R, Mefford I, *et al.* (1978). Lateralization of norepinephrine in human thalamus. *Science* 200: 1411–33.

Overlade DC. (1986). First aid for depression. In: Dowd ET, Healy JM, editors. *Case Studies in Hypnotherapy* (pp. 23–33). New York: Guilford Press.

Paykel ES, Meyers JK, Dienett MN, *et al.* P. (1969). Life events and depression: a controlled study. *Archives of General Psychiatry* 21: 753–60.

Paykel ES, Priest RG. (1992). Recognition and management of depression in general practice: Consensus Statement. *British Medical Journal* 305: 1198–202.

Pearlstein T, Stone A, Lund S, *et al.* (1997). Comparison of fluoxetine, bupropion, and placebo in the treatment of premenstrual dysphoric disorder. *Journal of Clinical Psychopharmacology* 17: 261–6.

Pincus HA, Pettit AR. (2001). The societal costs of chronic major depression. *Journal of Clinical Psychiatry* 62(Suppl. 6): 5–9.

Posner M. (1973). Coordination on internal codes. In: Chase W, editor. *Visual Information Processing*. New York: Academic Press.

Robins LN, Regier DA, editors. (1991). *Psychiatric Disorders in America: the Epidemiologic Catchment Area Study*. New York: Free Press.

Safer MA, Leventhal H. (1977). Ear differences in evaluating emotional tone of voice and verbal content. *Journal of Experimental Psychology: Human Perception and Performance* 3: 75–82.

Satcher D. (2000). Mental health: a report of the Surgeon General – executive summary. *Professional Psychology: Research and Practice* 31(1): 5–13.

Schoenberger NE. (2000). Research on hypnosis as an adjunct to cognitive-behavioral psychotherapy. *International Journal of Clinical and Experimental Hypnosis* 48: 154–69.

Schultz KD. (1978). Imagery and the control of depression. In: Singer Jl, Pope KS, editors. *The Power of Human Imagination: new methods in psychotherapy* (pp. 281–307). New York: Plenum Press.

Schultz KD. (1984). The use of imagery in alleviating depression. In: Sheik AA, editor. *Imagination and Healing* (pp. 129–58). New York: Baywoood Publishing Co. Inc.

Schultz KD. (2003). The use of imagery in alleviating depression. In: Sheikh AA, editor. *Healing Images: the role of imagination in health* (pp. 343–80). New York: Baywood Publishing Company, Inc.

Schwartz G. (1976). Facial muscle patterning in affective imagery in depressed and non-depressed subjects. *Science* 192: 489.

Schwartz G. (1977). Psychosomatic disorders in biofeedback: a psychological model of disregulation. In: Maser JD, Seligman MEP, editors. *Psychopathology: experimental models* (pp. 270–307). San Francisco: WH Freeman.

Schwartz G. (1984). Psychophysiology of imagery and healing: a systems perspective. In: Sheik AA, editor. *Imagination and Healing* (pp. 35–50). New York: Baywood Publishing Co. Inc.

Seligman MEP. (1975). *Helplessness: on depression, development of death*. San Francisco: WH Freeman.

Shevrin H. (1978). Evoked potential evidence for unconscious mental process: a review of the literature. In: Prangishvilli AS, Sherozia AE, Bassin FV, editors. *The Unconscious: nature, functions, methods of study*. Tbilisi, USSR: Metsnierba.

Shevrin H, Dickman, S. (1980). The psychologically unconscious American. *American Psychologist* 5: 421.

Simons AD, Garfield SL, Murphy, GE. (1984). The process of change in cognitive therapy and pharmacotherapy for depression. *Archives of General Psychiatry* 41: 45–51.

Solomon DA, Keller MB, Leon AC, *et al.* (2000). Multiple recurrences of major depressive disorder. *American Journal of Psychiatry* 157(2): 229–33.

Starker S, Singer JL. (1975). Daydreaming patterns of self-awareness in psychiatric patients. *Journal of Nervous and Mental Disease* 161: 313–17.

Sternberg S. (1975). Memory scanning: new findings and current controversies. *Quarterly Journal of Experimental Psychology* 27: 1.

Thase ME, Beck AT. (1992). An overview of cognitive therapy. In: Wright JH, Thase ME, Beck AT, *et al. Cognitive Therapy with Inpatients: developing a cognitive milieu.* New York: Guilford Press.

Tosi DJ, Baisden BS. (1984). Cognitive-experiential therapy and hypnosis. In: Wester WC, Smith AH, editors. *Clinical Hypnosis: a multidisciplinary approach* (pp. 155–78). New York: JB Lippincott Co.

Traynor JD. (1974). *Patterns of Daydreaming and Their Relationship to Depressive Affect.* Unpublished master's thesis. Miami University, Oxford, Ohio.

Wade TJ, Cairney J. (2000). Major depressive disorder and marital transition among mothers: results from a national panel study. *Journal of Nervous and Mental Disease* 188: 741–50.

Warren WL. (1994). *Revised Hamilton Rating Scale for Depression (RHRSD): manual.* Los Angeles: Western Psychological Services.

Weissman A, Beck AT. (1978). *Development and Validation of the Dysfunctional Attitude Scale.* Paper presented at the annual meeting for the Association for Advancement of Behavior Therapy, Chicago.

West LJ. (1967). Dissociative reaction. In: Freedman AM, Kaplan HI, editors. *Comprehensive Textbook of Psychiatry.* Baltimore, MD: Williams and Wilkins Co.

Williams JMG. (1992). *The Psychological Treatment of Depression.* London: Routledge.

Williams JMG, Watts FN, MacLeod C, *et al.* (1997). *Cognitive Psychology and Emotional Disorders.* Chichester, UK: Wiley.

World Health Organization (1992). *The ICD-10: the ICD-10 classification of mental and behavioral disorders: clinical descriptions and diagnostic guidelines.* Geneva: World Health Organization.

World Health Organization (1998). *Well-being Measures in Primary Healthcare/The Depcare Project.* Copenhagen: WHO Regional Office for Europe.

Yapko MD. (1992). *Hypnosis and the Treatment of Depressions: strategies for change.* New York: Brunner/Mazel Publishers.

Yapko MD. (2001). *Treating Depression with Hypnosis: integrating cognitive-behavioral and strategic approaches.* Philadelphia, PA: Brunner/Rotledge.

Young AR, Beitchman JH. (2001). Learning disorders. In: Gabbard GO, editor. *Treatment of Psychiatric Disorders* (vol.1). 3rd ed. (pp. 109–24). Washington, DC: American Psychiatric Publishing.

Youngren MA, Lewinshon PM. (1980). The functional relation between depression and problematic interpersonal behaviour. *Journal of Abnormal Psychology* 89: 333–41.

Zarren J, Eimer B. (2001). *Brief Cognitive Hypnosis: facilitating the change of dysfunctional behavior.* New York: Springer.

CHAPTER 6

Training in Hypnotherapy

Most of the professional organizations listed below provide excellent training in introductory, intermediate and advanced clinical hypnosis to qualified professionals. The Canadian Federation of Clinical Hypnosis describes the three levels of clinical hypnosis training as follows (*see*: http://www.clinicalhypnosis.ca).

Introductory workshops teach the basic required skills and knowledge of clinical hypnosis. They almost always involve 20 hours of training, and completion of the course is required both for membership and in order to take additional courses.

Intermediate courses deal more in specific content areas and provide an opportunity for supervised practice. They form an excellent stepping-stone in the integration of hypnotherapeutic techniques with your usual practice. You can expect to see intermediate courses dealing with issues such as pain management, anxiety, depression, psychosomatic disorders and ethics. You must take an introductory program prior to taking intermediate courses.

Advanced courses deal with specific topics (pain management, psychosomatics, anxiety, palliative care, medical procedures, etc.) and assume a basic knowledge and some extended experience/skill on the part of the learner.

By 'qualified professionals' most professional organizations imply professionals with licensure or registration in a healthcare profession. For example, the American Society of Clinical Hypnosis (ASCH) states (*see*: http://www. asch.net):

> To be eligible for **Full Membership** in ASCH, applicants must hold a doctorate in medicine (MD or DO), dentistry, podiatry (DPM), chiropractic, or psychology, or an equivalent doctoral degree with psychology as the major field of study,

or a masters level degree in nursing, social work, psychology, speech-language pathology, counseling, or marital/family therapy. In addition, applicants must be licensed or certified in the state in which they practice, be a member of a professional society consistent with their degree, such as the AMA, APA or ADA, have a stated interest in the clinical use of hypnosis, and have completed twenty hours of ASCH approved training in clinical hypnosis.

Associate Membership is for people who meet all the above criteria except the twenty hours of training. Associate Members have two years to meet the training requirement after joining.

Students enrolled in doctoral programs in medicine, dentistry, podiatry or psychology, or masters level programs in nursing, social work, psychology, or marital/family therapy, are eligible for **Student Affiliate** status at a reduced rate.

Resident/Intern Affiliate Status is available for full time residents or interns participating in a recognized medical, dental, podiatric or psychological residency or internship program.

A special category of membership is now available for individuals engaged in full time research and teaching related to clinical hypnosis at an accredited university or other institution of higher learning, or engaged full time in research related to clinical hypnosis at a governmental or research agency. For more information, please contact Dana Downing, Member Services Manager, at dhdowning@asch.net or by phone at 630/980-4740.

Many non-professional organizations offer training in hypnosis, but these courses may not meet the requirement for membership in a professional organization. It is advisable to consult with the organization you wish to join before enrolling in a hypnosis training program. The American Society of Clinical Hypnosis (ASCH) also provides certification and approved consultant programs, as described in its web page (*see*: http://www.asch.net):

> Certification offers non-statutory voluntary credentialing in Clinical Hypnosis and provides recognition of the advanced clinician who has met educational qualifications and required training in clinical hypnosis. The **ASCH Certification and Approved Consultant Program** is gaining national recognition as a standard for the practice of hypnosis. Anecdotal evidence suggests that hospitals and third party payers are beginning to recognize the importance of such standards and view ASCH Certification as a basic requirement for promoting hypnosis as a treatment modality.

What Certification Indicates

Certification does not automatically imply competence or guarantee the quality of a practitioner's work. Certification does indicate several things that fellow professionals, consumers, third party payers, managed care programs, hospitals and clinics are all interested in knowing about individuals who incorporate hypnosis in their practices. Certification indicates that the practitioner:

1. has undergone advanced training in his/her profession to obtain a legitimate advanced degree from an accredited institution of higher education
2. is licensed or certified to practice in his/her state/province
3. has had his/her education and training in clinical hypnosis reviewed by qualified peers and approved consultants and such training has met the minimum requirements established by a Standards of Training Committee of qualified peers
4. has been determined to have received at least the minimum educational training that ASCH, the largest such interdisciplinary organization in North America, considers as necessary for utilizing hypnosis.

LEVELS OF CERTIFICATION

There are two (2) levels of certification. Entry level is simply called 'Certification'. An advanced level, called 'Approved Consultant', recognizes individuals who have obtained advanced training in clinical hypnosis and who have extensive experience in utilizing hypnosis within their professional practices. Approved Consultants are qualified to provide individualized training and consultation for those seeking certification.

HOW ASCH CERTIFICATION DIFFERS FROM OTHER CERTIFICATION PROGRAMS

ASCH Certification in Clinical Hypnosis is distinct from other 'certification' programs in that it ensures that the certified individual is a bona fide health care professional who is licensed in his or her state or province to provide medical, dental, or psychotherapeutic services. ASCH believes that persons trained only in hypnosis lack the diagnostic and therapeutic skills as well as the licensure required to safely and responsibly treat medical, psychological, or dental problems with hypnosis. ASCH Certification distinguishes the professional practitioner from the lay hypnotist.

Certified professionals are encouraged to work toward attaining the highest level of advanced specialty certification in hypnosis through obtaining Diplomate Status from either the American Board of Medical Hypnosis, the American Board of Psychological Hypnosis, the American Board of Hypnosis in Dentistry, or the American Hypnosis Board for Clinical Social Work.

Requirements for Certification in Clinical Hypnosis

- MD, DDS, DMD, DO, DPM, PhD, PsyD, or equivalent doctoral degree with psychology as the major study, or a masters degree in nursing, social work, psychology, counseling, marriage and family therapy from a college or university accredited by its appropriate regional accrediting body
- membership in a professional society consistent with degree
- licensure or Certification by the state of province in which you practice
- minimum of 40 hours of ASCH approved workshop training (20 hours each of beginning and intermediate workshops)
- minimum of 20 hours of individualized training/consultation with an ASCH Approved Consultant
- minimum of two years of independent practice utilizing clinical hypnosis.

Requirements for Approved Consultant in Clinical Hypnosis

All of the above requirements, plus:

- minimum of 60 additional hours of ASCH approved workshop training
- minimum of five years of independent practice utilizing clinical hypnosis
- minimum of five years of membership in ASCH, SCEH, or equivalent.
- For Certification or Certification as an Approved Consultant applications, please see below or contact the ASCH office by fax (630/351-8490), phone (630/980-4740), or in writing at 140 N. Bloomingdale Rd., Bloomingdale, IL 60108-1017.

ADDRESSES AND WEBSITES OF PROFESSIONAL ORGANIZATIONS OF HYPNOSIS

There are several major national and international scientific professional societies of hypnosis. Some of the well-known societies are listed below. The list is not intended to be exhaustive.

American Psychological Association Division 30 – The Society of Psychological Hypnosis
750 First Street, NE
Washington, DC 20002-4242
USA
Phone: +1 800 374 2721, +1 202 336 5500, +1 202 336 6013
TDD: +1 202 218 6123
Fax: +1 202 218 3599
Publications:
  International Journal of Clinical and Experimental Hypnosis, official journal of the Society of Psychological Hypnosis
  Psychological Hypnosis, the quarterly newsletter of the Society.

American Society of Clinical Hypnosis (ASCH)
140 N. Bloomingdale Rd
Bloomingdale, IL 60108
USA
Phone: +1 630 980 740
Fax: +1 630 351 490
E-mail: info@asch.net
Website: http://www.asch.net/
Publications:
  American Journal of Clinical Hypnosis (ASCH) (see information for the American Society of Clinical Hypnosis).
  Editor: Stephen Lankton, MSW, DAHB
  Newsletter of the American Society of Clinical Hypnosis (quarterly)

Association Francaise d'Hypnotherapie
34 Rue des Guipons
94800 Villejuif
France
Email: becchio@club-internet.fr
Website: www.afhyp.com

Associazione Medica Italiana per lo Studio dell Ipnosi (AMISI)
Email: amisi@virgilio.it
Website: www.amisi.it

Australian Society of Hypnosis (ASH)
Victoria Branch, ASH
PO Box 5114,
Alphington, VIC 3078
Australia
Phone: +61 3 9499 5608
Fax: +61 3 9499 5806
Email: hypnosis@alphalink.com.au
Website: www.ozhypnosis.com.au
Publications:
    Australian Journal of Clinical and Experimental Hypnosis
    Website: www.ozhypnosis.com.au/journal/journal.htm

British Association of Medical Hypnosis (BAMH)
Suite 296
28 Old Brompton Road
London SW7 3SS
England
Phone: +44 208 998 4436
Email: secretary@bamh.org.uk
Website: http://www.hypnoforum.com/bamh/

British Society of Clinical Hypnosis (BSCH)
Organizing Secretary
125 Queensgate
Bridlington
East Yorkshire Y016 7JQ
Phone: +44 126 240103
Email: sec@bsch.org.uk
Website: http://www.bsch.org.uk/

British Society of Experimental and Clinical Hypnosis (BSECH)
National Office Secretary
28 Dale Park Gardens
Cookridge
Leeds LS16 7PT
England
Phone/fax: 07000 560309

Email: honsec@bsech.com
Website: http://www.bsech.com
Publications:
  Contemporary Hypnosis
  Editor: John Gruzelier

British Society of Medical and Dental Hypnosis (BSMDH)
28 Dale Park Gardens
Cookridge, Leeds
LS16 7PT
UK
Phone/fax: 07000 560309
Email: nat.office@bsmdh.org
Website: http://www.bsmdh.org

Canadian Federation of Clinical Hypnosis (CFCH)
Website: www.clinicalhypnosis.ca
The Canadian Federation of Clinical Hypnosis (CFCH) is the newly formed
national Canadian organization. It is the umbrella organization of its four
member provincial divisions (Alberta, Ontario, Quebec and Nova Scotia), to
which all current members belong. CFCH serves the interests of all four of its
provincial/regional organizations. Membership in CFCH occurs as a result
of achieving full membership in one or more of the provincial or regional
societies. You can navigate to the provincial/regional sites by going to 'CFCH
Provincial Societies' and directing questions accordingly.

Centro Ericksoniano de Mexico (CEM)
Email: cemenlinea@hipnosis.com.mx.
Website: http://centroericksoniano.edu.mx/

Centro Italiano Ipnosi Clinico-Sperimentale (CIICS)
Email: ciis@seleneweb.com

Centro Studi de Ipnosi Clinica e Psicoterapia 'H.Bernheim' (CSICHB)
Italy
Email: dirsan@villarosa.it

Dansk Selskab for Klinisk Hypnose (DSKH)
Website: www.hypnoterapi.com

**Deutsche Gesellschaft für Ärztliche Hypnose und Autogenes Trainig E.V.
(DGAHAT)**
Sekretariat
Posfach 1365
41463 Neuss
Germany
Website: http://web2.cylex.de/firma-home/deutsche-gesellschaft-fuer-aerztliche-
hypnose-und-autogenes-training--dgaehat--e-v--2081958.html

Deutsche Gesellschaft für Hypnose und Hypnotherapie
Email: DGH-Geschaeftsstellet@t-online.de
Website: http://dgh-hypnose.de/con/home
Publications:
> *Experimentelle und Klinische Hypnose*; Zeitschrift für Hypnose und
> Hypnotherapie

Deutsche Gesellschaft für Zahnärztliche Hypnose (DGZH)
Esslinger Str. 40
70182 Stuttgart
Germany
Email: mail@dgzh.de
Website: www.dgzh.de

European Society of Hypnosis (ESH)
PO Box 3352
Sheffield
S20 6WY
England
Phone: +44 114 247 4392
Fax: +44 114 247 4627
Email: mail@esh-hypnosis.org
Website: www.esh-hypnosis.de/
Publication:
> *European Journal of Clinical Hypnosis* (EJCH)

Hungarian Association of Hypnosis (HAH)
Email: mhesecretary@hotmail.com or GGACS@IZABELL.ELTE.HU
Magyar Hipnózis Egyesület
Website: www.hipnozis-mhe.hu

Hypnosis Society of New Zealand (NZSH)
PO Box 5015
Palmerston North
Phone: +64 9 376 0423
Email: katem@adhb.govt.nz
Website: http:/www.opotiki.com/hypnosisnz/

Indian Society of Clinical and Experimental Hypnosis (ISCEH)
Email: mrs_shovajana@im.eth.net

International Society of Hypnosis (ISH)
ISH Central Office
University Medical Center Utrecht
c/o PO Box 342
4000 AH Tiel
The Netherlands
Phone: +31 344 615427
Email: info@ish.web.org
Website: www.ish-web.org

Israel Society of Hypnosis (IsSH)
Email: info@hypno.org.il
Website: www.hypno.co.il/english.asp

Japan Institute of Hypnosis (JSH)
Email: saimin@kyorin-u.ac.jp
Website: www.j-hypno.com/

MEG: Milton H. Erickson Gesellschaft fur Klinische Hypnose E.V.
Waisenhausstrasse 55
80637 Munich
Germany
Website: www.MEG-hypnose.de

Publication:
Hypnose und Kognition

Nederlandse vereniging voor hypnose
Postbus 96
4000 AB TIEL
The Netherlands
Email: secretariaat@nvvh.com
Website: http://www.nvvh.com

Norsk Forening for Klinisk og Ekspeimental Hypnose
Email: guro@smerteklinikken.com
Website: www.hypnoseforeningen.no

ÖGATAP: Österreichische Gesellschaft fur Angewandt Tiefenpsychologie und Allgemeine Psychotherapie OGATAT Secretariat
Kaiserstr. 14/13
A-1070 Vienna
Austria
Email: office@oegatap.at
Website: www.oegatap.at

Sociedade Brasileira de Hipnose e Hipniatria
Email: sbhh@sbhh.org.br
Website: www.sbhh.org.br/sbhh/index.htm

Société d'Hypnose clinique Suisse (SHypS)
Email: ghyps@bluewin.ch
Website: www.hypnos.ch

Société Médicale Suisse d'Hypnose (SMSH)
Email: vrenigreising@csi.com
Website: www.smsh.ch

Societe Quebecoise d'Hypnose i (SQH)
Email: info@sqh.info
Website: www.sqh.info/

Society for Clinical and Experimental Hypnosis (SCEH)
Massachusetts School of Professional Psychology
221 Rivermoor Street
Boston, MA 02132
USA
Phone: +1 617 4691981
Email: sceh@mspp.edu
Website: www.sceh.us/
Publications:
    International Journal of Clinical and Experimental Hypnosis
    Website: www.ijceh.com/

South African Society of Clinical Hypnosis (SASCH)
Email: sasch@janopperman.com
Website: www.sasch.co.za/sasch/index.htm

Swedish Society of Clinical and Experimental Hypnosis (SSCEH)
SFKH's Kansli,
Flat 3,
s-931 85 Skelleftea
Sweden
Email: ssceh@telia.com

Tieteellinen Hypnoosi ri
Kylatie 8 M 6
16300 Orimattila
Finland
Email: admin@hypnoosi.net
Website: www.hypnoosi.net

Vlaams Wetenschappelijke Hypnose Vereniging
Email: VHYP@skynet.be
Website: www.vhyp.be/index.html

Index

Printed and bound by CPI Group (UK) Ltd, Croydon, CR0 4YY

23/10/2024

01777678-0015